Praise for

THE ELIMINATION DIET

"I've seen time and time again how eating the wrong foods can cause weight gain and fatigue. THE ELIMINATION DIET makes it easy to pinpoint what foods work best for you—this book is a life changer!"

—JJ Virgin, CNS, CHFS, *New York Times* bestselling author of *The Virgin Diet* and *JJ Virgin's Sugar Impact Diet*

"The most well-explained and evidence-based elimination diet that I have seen. I would highly recommend the program outlined in THE ELIMINA-TION DIET for anyone struggling with unexplained symptoms of anxiety, chronic pain, or poor digestion."

—Alan Christianson, NMD, author of *The Adrenal Reset Diet*, and founder, Integrative Health

Also by Alissa Segersten and Tom Malterre, MS, CN

The Whole Life Nutrition Cookbook

the ELIMINATION DIET

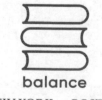

DISCOVER THE FOODS
THAT ARE MAKING
YOU SICK AND TIRED—
AND FEEL BETTER FAST

ALISSA SEGERSTEN AND
TOM MALTERRE, MS, CN

Foreword by Jeffrey Bland, Ph.D.

balance

NEW YORK • BOSTON

Copyright © 2015 by Whole Life Nutrition
Foreword copyright © 2015 by Jeffrey Bland, Ph.D.

Cover design by Tom McKeveny. Cover copyright © 2016 by Hachette Book Group, Inc.

Balance
Hachette Book Group
1290 Avenue of the Americas
New York, NY 10104
grandcentralpublishing.com
twitter.com/grandcentralpub

Originally published in hardcover and ebook by Grand Central Life & Style in March 2015
First Trade Paperback Edition: October 2016

Balance is an imprint of Grand Central Publishing. The Balance name and logo is a trademark of Hachette Book Group, Inc.

The Hachette Speakers Bureau provides a wide range of authors for speaking events. To find out more, go to www.HachetteSpeakersBureau.com or call (866) 376-6591.

The publisher is not responsible for websites (or their content) that are not owned by the publisher.

The Library of Congress has Cataloged the hardcover as follows:

Segersten, Alissa.
    The elimination diet : discover the foods that are making you sick and tired—and feel better fast / Alissa Segersten and Tom Malterre, MS, CN ; foreword by Jeffrey Bland.
        pages cm
Includes bibliographical references and index.
    ISBN 978-1-4555-8188-7 (hardback) — ISBN 978-1-4789-8747-5 (audio download) — ISBN 978-1-4555-8187-0 (ebook) — ISBN 978-1-4555-8186-3 (trade paperback)   1. Diet therapy.   2. Nutrition.   3. Cooking for the sick.   4. Detoxification (Health)   5. Food allergy—Diet therapy.   I. Malterre, Tom   II. Segersten, Alissa.   III. Title.
    RM216.S443 2015
    613.2—dc23
                                                                    2014048477

ISBNs: 978-1-4555-8186-3 (trade paperback), 978-1-4555-8187-0 (ebook)

Printed in the United States of America

LSC-C

Printing 7, 2022

To everyone suffering unnecessarily because they have not yet found the triggers that are contributing to their state of disease. May this book bring you the answers and the health you deserve.

ACKNOWLEDGMENTS

Above all, I have to thank my beautiful children. Their twinkling eyes and boundless energy give me hope for a bright future, and inspire me to do everything I can to assure that they have one.

I have to thank my heroes, idols, mentors, teachers, colleagues, and friends for all the incredible books, research papers, lectures, and recordings they have put out over the years that have completely changed my life and my practice.

Dr. John McDougall, my family doctor, inspired me to see food as the most powerful medicine on the planet.

Dr. Jeffrey Bland, Dr. Alan Gaby, Dr. Joe Pizzorno, Dr. Jonathan Wright, Dr. Leo Galland, and Dr. Mark Hyman taught me to look to food reactions as a primary contributor to diseases of the modern world.

Dr. Stephen Genuis, Dr. Walter Crinnion, Dr. Raymond Palmer, and Dr. Claudia Miller helped me to see the connection between our environmental exposures and the drastic rise in disease.

Dr. Don Huber, Dr. Michael Antoniou, and Jeffrey Smith have been extremely generous with their time and information in raising my awareness regarding genetically modified organisms and the pesticides associated with them.

Dr. Rodney Dietert, Dr. Sidney Baker, and Dr. Alessio Fasano helped to tie together all the loose ends in how food reactions, microorganisms, nutrient deficiencies, and environmental chemical exposures have all intertwined to give us the drastic rise of diseases and disorders we are seeing today.

Julie Matthews, CNC, Dr. Tom O'Bryan, Dr. Stephen Wangen, and Pamela Ferro, RN, ASN, have reaffirmed that clinical practices revolving around food sensitivity reactions are not only incredibly effective at helping clients, but are rewarding beyond imagination.

To Gretchen Lees, my wordsmith friend who helped me simplify my ideas to make this book a reality, a special heartfelt thanks for your skill, patience, and perseverance. And last but not least, I have to thank Ali for making all the science come together with simple, beautiful, incredible-tasting recipes, which are the true magic of this program and countless others.

—*Tom Malterre*

First and foremost, I would like to acknowledge my five children for being on the front line of taste-testing all of my new recipes. They have always given me their honest opinion on what they liked and what they didn't.

I'd like to thank all of my friends and family who tested and retested the recipes within these pages; I could never have completed this without your honest feedback and suggestions for new recipes. Specifically, I'd like to acknowledge Candace Allen, Jenna Anderson, and my mother, Deb Segersten, for their endless amount of recipe testing—you ladies are amazing!

We would like to thank Celeste Fine, our amazing literary agent, for keeping us on track and believing in us. We would also like to extend deep gratitude to our editor, Sarah Pelz from Grand Central Publishing, for making sure the science and information within these pages was accessible to all reading audiences.

And last, I would like to thank Tom for his breadth and depth of knowledge. His passion to understand complex scientific topics, so he can change the world for the better, inspires me every day to develop new recipes that will help people feel better and enjoy a more fulfilled life.

—*Alissa Segersten*

CONTENTS

FOREWORD

Food is supposed to be our friend. It nourishes us. It is part of the art of living. It connects us to the earth. It provides the building blocks that make up our body. In essence, food and the process of eating it represent one of the most important shared human experiences.

So, with that said, why do we have so much trouble with food? Why does it occupy so much of our conversation? Why does it seem at times to be our enemy?

In Tom Malterre and Alissa Segersten's book *The Elimination Diet*, you learn the good, bad, and ugly surrounding the relationship we have with our food. You will learn that the "food of one is the poison of another" based upon unique genetic responses to certain food substances like gluten and lactose. You will learn how our food has been adulterated by processing, "chemicalization," and contamination. You will learn that your body's immune system may recognize some food as a "foreign object" and will respond with a powerful "search and destroy" system that produces collateral damage, resulting in inflammation and increased risk of disease.

But more than this understanding of how food may react in your body, you will learn in this book of the beauty and power of good foods that are properly prepared and work with your unique body chemistry.

This occurs through an exploration of your individual food tolerances and intolerances, which you'll discover by following the Elimination Diet described in this book. From your experience in applying this program, you will learn how to eat the foods that make you healthy and avoid the foods that make you sick.

The story in this book goes well beyond the concept of a food allergy to describe the role that food and the substances in food have on the complex digestive, immune, and health and disease processes. It clearly describes why food can produce so many chronic symptoms—ranging from skin problems, to headaches and "foggy brain," to arthritis, and everything in between—that rob many people of their health and vitality.

This is a book written by a nutrition professional, Tom Malterre, who has counseled thousands of people on their diet. It is a book that teaches by case history and example. It is a book grounded in the latest nutritional concepts and discoveries that illuminate how important it is for our food to be compatible with our individual needs. This is a book that takes very complex topics on the relationship of food to our physiological function and makes them easy to understand. This is a book that will be a welcome relief for readers who have suffered for years with chronic health problems and are desperate for a solution.

But the book is more than that—in fact, it is two books in one. Thanks to Alissa Segersten, the later chapters feature one of the most remarkable recipe and menu planning tools you will ever find. The amazing recipes span a tremendous range of tasty, colorful, healthy, natural, and clean options for the reader who is ready to try the Elimination Diet. Having used many of these recipes for myself and my family, I can say with confidence that they deliver on the promise that good, clean foods can taste better than anything you have ever eaten.

For many people the issue is not the desire to improve their eating, but rather the challenge of how to do it successfully without becoming a food fanatic. The recipes and menu guides in the book are the key to taking the step from aspiration to action. You will find it fun to be introduced to so many new foods and fantastic ways of preparing them. It makes the Elimination Diet accessible and will help you achieve your goals of improving your health.

I have worked in the field of clinical nutrition for the past forty years. When we founded the Institute for Functional Medicine in 1991 to train health care practitioners on how to apply personalized lifestyle programs for their patients, we knew that diet, food, and nutrition were cornerstones in achieving optimal health. Tom Malterre and Alissa Segersten's *The Elimination Diet* takes the complex challenge of designing a personalized approach to food and makes it straightforward and simple enough that anyone motivated to make a positive change in their health can do it.

—Jeffrey Bland, Ph.D., FACN, Founder of the Institute for
Functional Medicine and Personalized Lifestyle
Medicine Institute; Author of *The Disease Delusion*

INTRODUCTION

I'm so excited you've picked up *The Elimination Diet*. The program you will find here has been used to change the lives of thousands of people. It is designed to help you feel better, look better, and live better.

The Elimination Diet is not your average diet. It's not about calories, fats, carbs, or portion control. It's not about depriving yourself of your favorite foods or punishing yourself. It's about creating a new awareness of how the foods you eat make you feel.

Whether you're aware of it or not, what you eat every day directly determines how you feel. Some foods can drag you down, make you sick, and create nagging pain, digestive discomfort…and more. You may not even realize all of the different ways food has been affecting you—you may think your fatigue, or brain fog, or joint pain, or heartburn, or even weight gain are normal for you. But that's far from the truth. These symptoms can all be helped and even eliminated by changing your diet. Just as some foods cause issues, others can provide incredible health and energy, boost your metabolism, give you great skin, improve your mood, and increase longevity.

In this book, you will discover the plan you need for identifying which foods make you feel good and which foods make you feel bad. This direct and simple approach will give you powerful control over your health.

I've been using the Elimination Diet in my clinical practice for more than ten years. The program has evolved over time as research and results have helped make the plan even more effective. The program in this book has been fine-tuned over the years to help my clients, my family, and even myself. In fact, my first discovery of it was by way of an experiment on my own health.

A DIET THAT CHANGED MY LIFE

I know what it's like to feel uncomfortable in your own body. In high school and throughout college, I would experience episodes of nagging joint pain, severe digestive discomfort, and dulling mental fog. In other words, I would go from being happy and sharp as a tack to grumpy, tired, and dealing with a miserably aching gut. What was most frustrating was the unpredictability—I never really knew when these flu-like symptoms were going to hit me or what was causing them.

While in school for my master's degree, I went on a raw food detox diet for a few weeks, and the muddy thoughts in my head cleared up, the nagging joint pain disappeared, I had boundless energy, and my digestive troubles normalized.

I was amazed at how much better I felt. But it didn't last. As soon as I went back to eating my favorite staples like sourdough rye bread and whole wheat tortillas, the agony returned immediately. I knew I had found the source of my symptoms: gluten. When I took the gluten out for good, my entire life got lifted to a new level I never even dreamed was possible.

Even though I didn't realize it at the time, this self-experiment was my first experience with an elimination diet. By removing foods and then adding them back in, I was able to determine which foods were causing my symptoms. It was a profound and life-changing discovery—it put me in control of my health.

I started to explore elimination diets further. I had learned about their history and use from Dr. Alan Gaby, former president of the American Holistic Medicine Association, and Dr. Joe Pizzorno, coauthor of the *Encyclopedia of Natural Medicine*. After reviewing my notes from their lectures and literature, and evaluating numerous research articles, it became clear that this was a potent and proven tool that should be used by all nutritionists. Pretty soon I was convincing all my friends, family, and acquaintances to try the Elimination Diet. Some of the results were close to miraculous, as joint pain, fatigue, and headaches all but disappeared.

Completely blown away by the power of this simple intervention, I opened my own clinical practice and started telling clients that they would feel fantastic if they could just cut out foods like gluten, dairy, eggs, yeast, soy, and corn for 28 days. I was met with the same simple question over and over again. "Ummm...so what do I eat?"

Thankfully, I had a secret weapon: Ali Segersten. Ali, a fellow graduate of the Bastyr University nutrition program and the coauthor of this book, is a recipe-making genius! I have literally never met another human who can invent more delicious, wholesome, and gorgeous recipes than her. (I'm lucky: She's my wife, too.)

Ali would take any request—no matter how challenging—and come up with an elimination diet–friendly recipe. My clients were ecstatic with the results and I would print off stacks of recipes at the end of my appointments. They were huge hits! Everyone was amazed at how delicious eating this way could be.

It wasn't long before we had hundreds of requests to put together a cook-book with Elimination Diet–friendly recipes. In 2006, we self-published the *Whole Life Nutrition Cookbook*, which contained a condensed and simplified version of the Elimination Diet. After ordering a thousand copies, we were sure that our pallet of books would gather dust in our garage for years. But we sold more than 400 copies in just a few weeks, and within a few months we were completely sold out. Both clients and practitioners were scrambling for copies to share with their friends and families. Within a few years, the gluten-free trend took off and our cookbook became a cult classic in the Northwest and among Functional Medicine practitioners across the United States and Canada. More than 60,000 copies and ten years later, Ali's recipes are still winning over the hearts and taste buds of people around the globe.

We've also used our websites, WholeLifeNutrition.net and Nourishing Meals.com, to share how-to and informative videos, new recipes, and over-views of many of the concepts that are introduced in our books and within my practice. If you want additional resources, like helpful videos or cook-ing demos, visit the Elimination Diet page on our site, which provides extra resources to help you succeed while participating in this life-changing process.

The Elimination Diet is without a doubt the clear cornerstone of the work I do in my practice. Through my practice and our websites, we've used it to help thousands of people eliminate migraines, digestive issues, skin prob-lems, joint pain, unwanted weight gain, fatigue, and more.

And now we're bringing it to you in this book. Are you ready to improve your life and finally create freedom from unnecessary symptoms? It's all within your reach.

HOW TO USE THIS BOOK

In Part 1, you'll read about the core concepts of the Elimination Diet, and discover why it's so important to use food first to let go of your symptoms. You'll also learn about the glorious gut and why normal digestive functions are so important to your complete health. Plus, you will learn about the most common foods linked to food reactions, and how environmental triggers might be hurting your health.

Part 2 will get you excited and prepared to start the Elimination Diet. You'll find great ideas and strategies for reducing stress, improving metabolism, managing detox systems, and preparing yourself mentally for the program. Don't miss this section! Plenty of the action items can be implemented immediately and will help move you toward feeling better right away. Included here are essential kitchen items you'll need during the diet and a complete shopping list for when you're ready to hit the store.

In Part 3, you will find the three phases of the Elimination Diet laid out for you in detail. We've included sample meal plans for each phase, complete "yes" and "no" food lists so you know exactly what to include and exclude, and information on how to pick the best foods for feeling great. In chapter 11, you'll hear directly from Ali as she shares with you an incredible number of recipes for all three phases of the program. Get ready to explore the delicious and rejuvenating world of fresh, whole, healing foods. You'll also find here a chapter on special dietary considerations and commonly asked questions.

Be sure to also check out the Resources section for info on where to find many of our recommended products and a selection of research studies that support the content of this book.

IT'S YOUR TURN

On the pages that follow, you will discover all the steps you need to take to feel great: which foods to remove, which to keep, and which foods and supplements to add; hundreds of delicious, easy to make recipes; and support and inspiration to ensure your success.

This book was written to help you feel better. There is too much unnecessary suffering in the world today. After seeing thousands of people wake up to new lives full of passion, joy, and vibrant health, I have made it my mission to share this process with as many people as possible. Life is short. Live it to the fullest!

PART I

Why the
Elimination Diet Works

1

FOOD IS THE MOST POWERFUL TOOL FOR CHANGING YOUR LIFE

Whether you have experienced the power of food yourself or know one of the millions of people who have changed their diet and healed themselves, from stomach upset, migraines, eczema, unexplained weight gain, or chronic fatigue, you have a feeling this diet will help you. Chances are, you are right.

After lecturing across the United States and Canada, seeing thousands of clients in clinical practice over the last decade, and earning two degrees in nutritional sciences, I have seen no other thing help people more than the Elimination Diet. They can be at the end of all hope, seeing numerous specialists and taking countless medications, and come back from the brink. All by changing their food.

CASE STUDY

In 2006, Sally came to me as what I can accurately describe as a mere shell of a human being. She shuffled into my office with her head hanging low, leaning on her husband for support. When Sally spoke, there was no emotion behind her voice. No passion. No energy. Her fatigue was so extreme that she had a difficult time holding her head up to look at me during our conversation. Her husband told me that she was lucky to have 5 hours in a day that she was awake enough to function. It was obvious that her life-force was severely depleted.

Sally's medical file was as thick as an encyclopedia. She was in the care of six medical specialists for issues including constant stomach and bowel upset along with diarrhea, debilitating fatigue, breathing problems, sleep issues, and alternating anxiety and depression that left her completely dysfunctional. The "official" medical diagnoses had been atypical bipolar disorder, chronic fatigue, gastroesophageal reflux disease (GERD), irritable bowel syndrome, mitochondrial dysfunction, sleep apnea, asthma, and hypertension.

Whenever I see a case like this, I always know the first place to look: food. I knew right away that Sally needed the Elimination Diet. Eight out of ten times, it will be *the* factor that changes the course of my clients' health.

Sally had nothing to lose and everything to gain. She cleared her cupboards of all gluten-containing flours, donated bags of corn chips to the neighbors, started following simple meal plans, and began the cooking fest.

Within twelve days of starting the Elimination Diet, Sally woke up. It was as if she had been in and out of sleep for the last ten years and was finally fully awake. The color came back into her face. There was a spring in her step and emotion behind her voice. She went from a lifeless person to a 15-hour-a-day go-getter.

A few months later, the medical specialists were all in shock with her progress and slowly weaned Sally off of every one of her medications as she no longer fit the diagnostic criteria for *any* of her previous conditions. No irritable bowel. No anxiety or depression. No sleep apnea. No chronic fatigue. She did have one complaint, though: Sally had to buy a whole new wardrobe as her excess pounds melted away along with all her health conditions.

Sally quite literally changed her life by changing her diet. Through the Elimination Diet, she was able to discover that foods like gluten and soy brought on her fatigue and other symptoms. As long as she avoids these foods, she avoids her symptoms.

REMARKABLE RESULTS

Every day the Elimination Diet helps people like Sally feel good again. Some of the remarkable success I've seen in my own practice by changing food alone:

- Jim, 81, let go of arthritis pain
- Christy, 48, got rid of her migraines and back pain
- Penelope, 2, healed her intestines
- Marian, 58, let go of carpal tunnel syndrome and felt 20 years younger
- Joan, 42, had her eczema disappear
- Siblings Charles and Katie, 7 and 9 respectively, improved their autistic symptoms
- Daniel, 44, lost 30 pounds and lowered his blood pressure
- Julie, 17, stopped vomiting after meals
- Linda, 53, experienced clear thinking for the first time in years
- Alex, 25, let go of his embarrassing gas

. . . and the list goes on.

It doesn't matter if someone comes in with constipation, obesity, MS, or high blood pressure, doing the Elimination Diet drastically alters how their body functions. The results never cease to amaze me.

Logically, it makes sense. Certain foods are chock-full of potentially harmful particles that are not digested well and can easily confuse and excite your immune cells. When we remove these foods that are the most likely to irritate us, many diseases will calm down.

I am not the only one witnessing these profound results. For decades, researchers have been documenting the power of using food to improve a long list of conditions. Here are just a few examples:

- A study published in the journal *Clinical Allergy* revealed that 91 percent of rheumatoid arthritis sufferers benefited from eliminating foods such as grains, milk, nuts, beef, and eggs.
- Research published in *The Lancet* determined that 85 percent of migraine sufferers could become headache-free by following an elimination diet. Wheat, oranges, eggs, tea, coffee, chocolate, milk, and corn were some of the foods linked to migraines.

■ J. C. Breneman, a pioneer in the area of food allergy research, found that symptoms of gallbladder disease could be eliminated in 100 percent of the people who followed an Elimination Diet. This research, published in the *Annals of Allergy*, showed that eggs, pork, onions, fowl, milk, coffee, oranges, corn, nuts, and tomatoes could cause the vast majority of gallbladder irritation.

The Institute for Functional Medicine (IFM), the educational organization that has trained some of the most cutting-edge physicians practicing medicine today, teaches the importance of elimination diets in all of their training programs. (I was fortunate enough to study there as well.)

During one of their courses, I heard many statements from esteemed faculty about how eliminating problem foods can help patients heal. Dr. Catherine Willner, a neurologist with the Mayo Clinic, mentioned that her MS clients might benefit from the removal of gluten from their diet. Dr. Mark Hyman, author, clinician, and the current chairman of the IFM board of directors, shared that he had instructed his nutrition staff to put patients on an elimination diet *before* he would see them in his office. He claimed that 80 percent of them got so much better that he only had to do some fine-tuning from there.

And at another educational seminar, world-renowned thyroid expert and Phoenix-based naturopathic doctor Alan Christianson said that he had seen elimination diets completely change the course of his patients with certain types of thyroid disease.

All of these practitioners (and countless others) were seeing the same things as I was seeing in clinical practice. And why wouldn't they? Most of the common unnecessary symptoms plaguing people today are happening because something is irritating the body. And for more and more people, foods are the primary irritants.

IS YOUR BODY IRRITATED?

When your body is irritated, there is only one way it knows how to respond: It gets inflamed, and sends chemical messengers and immune cells to attack whatever is causing the irritation.

When this attack is going on within the body, symptoms such as fatigue, brain fog, and joint pain can be experienced. You might feel kind of like you're getting the flu, but the lousy feelings never really go away or they seem to come and go mysteriously.

What's likely going on is your body is fighting a battle every time you eat. It's possible that the foods you're eating are being mistaken for dangerous compounds like bacteria and viruses. Could that be why you are walking around with gut pain, brain fog, anxiety, headaches, back pain, and a few extra pounds? Yes. In fact, every common disease that people are suffering from has this inflamed state—better known as inflammation—at its core (you'll learn more about inflammation later in this chapter).

To create healing, we must look to food first. This is not a new concept, but rather a time- and research-tested approach to unnecessary and frustrating symptoms.

THE NEW OLD MEDICINE

Before the introduction of pharmaceuticals, doctors/teachers/medicine men/wise women from all corners of the earth knew that foods created a response in the body. They knew that certain foods promoted mucus, while others cleared it. They knew there were particular foods to avoid when you were feeling anxious, and others to eat to feel calm. And more important, they knew that each person reacted differently to all foods.

Even the designated father of western medicine, Hippocrates, famously stated: "Let thy food be thy medicine." And yet you'd be hard-pressed to find a practitioner of modern medicine who asks you the most basic question: What do you eat every day?

It baffles me that the most influential action we can take to improve our health is often ignored by modern medicine. We can change that with the Elimination Diet.

CASE STUDY

Malinda came to my office presenting with significant mood issues and feeling as if she was "falling apart." For the life of her, she could not calm down and get a good night's sleep because her anxiety was overwhelming. She had uterine fibroids and erratic bowel movements.

Like many of my clients, she was referred by a doctor, and had a very extensive medical history that included a lengthy list of symptoms, lab results, and plenty of medications. It told a story of years of significant physical and emotional pain.

Malinda had seen numerous specialists, but not one had been able to help her.

As part of every appointment, I do what is called a dietary intake, which means I asked her questions about what she ate and drank throughout a typical day. The conversation went something like this:

ME: What is the first thing you eat or drink when you wake up in the morning and what time is that?

MALINDA: Well, I wake up pretty early and have a soda around 6 a.m.

ME: And the next thing you either ate or drank?

MALINDA: Around 11 a.m. I would have another soda and maybe a saltine cracker.

ME: Is there anything else?

MALINDA: No.

ME: And your next food or drink?

MALINDA: I may have a soda and half of a chocolate bar around 2:30 or 3:00.

ME: Is there anything after that?

MALINDA: Yes. I will often have another soda right before dinner around 5:45 and maybe another cracker.

ME: What would you be eating for dinner?

MALINDA: Sometimes I will have a small piece of chicken and some salad. Other times I will eat half of a package of saltine crackers or the second half of my chocolate bar with another soda.

ME: Anything after that?

MALINDA: Maybe a small piece of chocolate and a soda. That's it.

ME: Is this a typical day for you?

MALINDA: Yes. I eat pretty much the same thing most days.

ME: How long have you been eating these same things?

MALINDA: For many years.

For years Malinda had been suffering, and for years not a single person had asked her what she was eating.

It is time we look to diet as being at the root of health and wellness in our society. And there is no better tool to examine the effect of our diet on our health than the Elimination Diet. Allergists have been using elimination diets for centuries to determine which harmful foods were causing severe breathing and skin conditions. More recently, Functional Medicine doctors have recognized that they play a much broader role in health care. The success they're reporting in treating autoimmune disorders, intestinal issues, and other chronic health conditions is helping the diet to finally get noticed by mainstream medicine.

I've been implementing this dietary program in my own practice for ten years to help people with laundry lists of symptoms. I have never seen anything produce greater and more profound changes in people's lives. More important, the changes happen fast: if not within the first few days, then within the first few weeks. Research articles reflect that others have seen these same speedy results.

The migraine study referenced earlier from *The Lancet* reported that headaches disappeared within the first five days in the majority of cases. The previously mentioned research of Dr. J. C. Breneman revealed that discomfort related to gallbladder disease improved within three to five days of starting an elimination diet. In "The effect of diet in rheumatoid arthritis," published in *Clinical and Experimental Allergy*, symptoms of rheumatoid arthritis were shown to improve after 10 days of eliminating trigger foods.

In my clinical nutrition practice, more than 80 percent of people who go on the Elimination Diet feel better. Within three to five days, many experience relief from symptoms they've dealt with for decades. Within twelve to fourteen days, they feel like they have a new lease on life. For a small investment of time, you can get a return of living life on a completely new level. Is it your turn to feel better?

THE BENEFITS OF
THE ELIMINATION DIET

Because I have been trained in Functional Medicine, the diet shared in this book is closely related to the diet recommended by the Institute for Functional Medicine. After reviewing hundreds of articles and getting feedback from thousands of participants, this updated diet has been designed to help the highest number of people suffering from a large range of disorders.

Both historical and modern texts were referenced, industry experts were interviewed, and countless scientific articles were read to determine which foods would be taken out and which foods would be added on the program found in this book.

Perhaps most important of all are the life-changing results of all the people who have gone before you. These individuals have paved the way to getting better fast, and they've experienced incredible benefits by following the Elimination Diet. Let's explore these real-life benefits a bit more and see what people have had to say about their experiences.

The Eight Benefits of the Elimination Diet

Benefit #1: A Clear Mind

Symptoms/conditions eliminated or reduced:

Foggy thinking
Short-term memory issues
Anxiety and hyperactivity
Symptoms of depression

In their own words:

"I feel like the fog has lifted!"
"My keys are not getting lost anymore."
"Our son has gone from bouncing off the walls to playing quietly."
"I actually want to get out of bed now."

Benefit #2: A Calm Gut

Symptoms/conditions eliminated or reduced:

Gas and bloating
Reflux (gastroesophageal reflux disease or GERD)
Diarrhea and constipation
Cramping and pain

In their own words:

"So these pants fit me after all! I was loosening my belt so much after eating that I was beginning to wonder."

"My wife thanks you profusely for putting me on this diet."

"I had no idea six or more bowel movements a day was not normal."

"I had no idea two bowel movements a week was not normal."

"Sitting at my desk for more than an hour before rushing to the bathroom probably saved my job."

"There are no more knives in my gut after I eat."

Benefit #3: No Pain

Symptoms/conditions eliminated or reduced:

Back pain

Arthritis

Leg cramps

Carpal tunnel

In their own words:

"I can't believe it. The doctors said I would suffer for the rest of my life."

"Not only is the pain in my back gone, but I can move more freely now."

"How is it that food changed my carpal tunnel? I thought that was a repetitive motion disorder?"

CASE STUDY

Marian, a busy, 58-year-old schoolteacher from California, called complaining of constant arthritis pain. She had been experiencing this pain for more than eight years and had heard that dietary changes may be able to help. Her other conditions also included carpal tunnel syndrome, trigger finger, frequent loose stools, and fatigue. After our initial phone consult, I suspected her symptoms indicated a potential sensitivity to gluten-containing foods. I recommended Marian try gluten elimination. After her initial two-week dietary change, her symptoms and pain diminished substantially, her bowel movements normalized, and she experienced increased energy. When she follows a gluten-free diet, she lives pain-free, and says she feels twenty years younger.

Benefit #4: Headache Free

Symptoms/conditions eliminated or reduced:

Headaches

Migraines

In their own words:

"I went from having 2 to 4 headaches a week to zero and it only took 5 days!"

"My migraines are completely controlled with Epsom baths and the elimination of certain foods."

CASE STUDY

Jeremy was a 10-year-old who was getting robbed of his childhood. Instead of going to school and playing with his friends every day, he was suffering from debilitating migraines 1 to 2 times per week. The headaches measured a 9 out of 10 on a pain scale, and some were so painful that he ended up in the hospital for treatment. The only way he could lessen the attacks was to lie in his darkened room with sunglasses on and take different supplements and medications, such as vitamin B2, magnesium, Tylenol, Advil, rizatriptan, Intuniv, and Depakote. Along with the head pain, he had stomach pains, and his mood was so bad that he had to see a psychiatrist after an outburst that left him in the emergency room. As with all other migraine cases, I knew exactly what to do: I suggested to Jeremy's mom that she change his diet immediately and have him begin taking Epsom salt baths. I gave her a list of the top eleven migraine-inducing foods—gluten, dairy, eggs, yeast, corn, sugar, citrus, tea, coffee, chocolate, and beef—and asked her to buy only organic foods.

Just three days later, I received an e-mail from Jeremy's mom asking, "Is it possible that we are already seeing results??? My son just told me that his headache has gone from a pain level of nine to seven/eight and his stomach down to a seven! This is the first relief he has had in weeks!"

By replacing his milk and fruit punch, pancakes and syrup, and pizza and chocolate milk with homemade chicken soup, sautéed kale, and smoothies, his pain was beginning to subside. His energy perked up and his mom said he was happier. After five days, the pain was gone. After seven days, his mood improved tremendously. On day 8, however, Jeremy ate some candy-coated nuts he found stashed somewhere and his moodiness came back with a vengeance. Within a few days of returning to the diet, he was back to feeling great. Jeremy now takes control of his mood and his migraines with every bite of food he eats.

Benefit #5: Better Breathing

Symptoms/conditions eliminated or reduced:

Asthma
Chronic rhinitis
Sinus congestion
Postnasal drip
Recurring sinus infections

In their own words:

"I was beginning to think this constant postnasal drip was genetic."
"I haven't had a single sinus infection since I found my food sensitivities."
"My daughter's asthma can be turned on and off with foods."

CASE STUDY

Joan was looking for some solutions for her 2-year-old daughter, Katie, who had severe asthma. Her doctor's skin-prick test had identified Katie as having multiple airborne allergies, including dust, mold, and pollen. The toddler also displayed behavioral problems, had dark circles under her eyes, and suffered from reoccurring sinus infections. After a few visits to the emergency room for some severe asthma attacks, Katie's family did everything they could to eliminate the airborne allergens in their home: They removed all of their carpeting and replaced it with hardwood flooring, repainted the walls, and covered all mattresses and pillows with hypoallergenic covers. Even after doing all of this, Katie's symptoms did not change. I suggested to Joan that Katie's symptoms might be associated with a dairy sensitivity. She was extremely resistant to hearing this because cheese was her daughter's favorite food—how could she deprive Katie of the one food she craved the most? But I believed what Katie was really being deprived of was her health. After a few more consultations and a health food store tour, Joan felt confident that she had enough dairy-free food options for her daughter. After two weeks of eating dairy-free, the asthma attacks stopped and Katie's sinuses began to drain—it took more than three days before they completely cleared up. For the first time since Joan could remember, Katie could breathe freely through her nose. And as long as Katie stayed dairy-free, her sinuses stayed clear and her asthma stayed away. Due to some intestinal complaints later on, Joan put Katie on a gluten-free diet and those cleared up as well.

Benefit #6: Clearer Skin

Symptoms/conditions eliminated or reduced:

Acne
Eczema
Atopic dermatitis
Psoriasis
Hives

In their own words:

"I have tried creams and medications but nothing would make this rash better. Who would have thought it was the food all along?"

"My skin got less red at first and then it started to heal. In three weeks' time it looked better than it has in years."

Benefit # 7: Increased Energy

Symptoms/conditions eliminated or reduced:

Chronic fatigue
Mild fatigue/low energy
Muscle weakness
Insomnia

In their own words:

"Before the Elimination Diet, it felt like I was walking through molasses all the time."
"Honestly, I think I was sleepwalking for the last 10 years."
"So this is what life is supposed to be like?! I love getting out of bed now!"

In case you missed it, turn back to page 3 to read about Sally's incredible recovery from chronic fatigue (and many other conditions).

Benefit #8: Weight Control

Symptoms/conditions eliminated or reduced:

Weight loss resistance
Trouble gaining weight

In their own words:

Overweight: "Cutting my calories didn't work. Cutting out carbs didn't work. Cutting out my reactive foods shed my pounds faster than I ever thought possible."

Underweight: "No matter how much I ate when my intestines were irritated, the pounds kept coming off. When I eat the right foods, I can eat less and still maintain a healthy weight."

If you don't see your particular symptom or condition listed here, don't worry—the Elimination Diet helps with several other issues; the benefits listed here are simply some of the most common I've witnessed within my clinic.

A PLAN TO MAKE YOU FEEL BETTER

Putting food at the center of your health care is surprisingly foreign to many. Avoiding many of the foods you are accustomed to eating is even stranger. Any new strategy needs a plan, a road map in how to navigate change. That's what this book is: a guide to show you why you need an Elimination Diet, what an Elimination Diet is, and how to do an Elimination Diet.

You are going to learn how to perform a simple experiment of removing foods, watching as your symptoms go away, and then adding foods back in to determine which ones may be contributing to your discomfort. This approach offers you the ultimate in diet customization; like a tailored dress or pair of pants, the diet you end up with will be ideal for your body and suit your unique personal needs.

In addition to removing some of the most common food irritants, we'll also work to increase the amount of healing and beneficial foods in your diet. These will help repair and replenish your tired cells. Having rejuvenated cells will improve your metabolism, energy levels, digestion, and appearance.

If you're like some of my clients, you've been trying to get to the bottom of your symptoms for years, maybe even decades. I understand the discomfort and the frustration that comes with the lack of answers—and I'm here to help guide you through this healing process.

Most important, I want you to know that you can get rid of joint pain, digestive problems, stubborn extra pounds, headaches, moodiness, skin rashes and irritation, low energy, and more. Once those disappear, you may be able to stop taking some medications that aren't working for you, and are possibly even making you feel worse.

The first step is to bring your focus to foods, but not in the typical way you might expect from a diet. As you explore this program, I want you to begin to create a new awareness of how foods make you feel. Start to really look at your meals and take note of your symptoms. If food is the most likely suspect in irritating your body and contributing to your symptoms, it is time to put your attention toward the foods you eat and how they are impacting your health.

You will be asked to think of the food you eat in a completely different way. Every bite you take can mean a step toward freedom from your suffering or a step back into pain. This is going to take some commitment and time on your part, but it will be so worth it when you have a customized diet and are free of the troubles that are plaguing you!

THE FOODS YOU EAT: THE PROBLEM AND THE SOLUTION

Food is powerful stuff—it can be both the poison that programs your body for discomfort and disease and the remedy that rejuvenates your cells and body systems. It can be the instigator of discomfort and disease or the cure for both.

When you eat processed foods, food additives, chemicals, artificial sweeteners, high-fructose corn syrup, and other inflammatory foods, you create a toxic, irritated environment. These foods and substances inflame the intestinal tract, which begins to simmer with heat like a hot bed of coals. As you continue to eat the same foods, the fire spreads through the whole body—and you've got system-wide inflammation. This type of inflammation is linked to allergies, heart disease, type 2 diabetes, high blood pressure, sleep apnea, and even depression.

But the Elimination Diet is not an anti-food program—quite the opposite. While conducting this simple experiment, you'll be eating lots of other foods that are incredibly healing, not to mention filling and delicious! These foods are rich in antioxidants, vitamins, and minerals. They're full of wonderful anti-inflammatory properties that help the body detoxify and heal. They repair and replenish cells, improving energy and metabolism and maximizing health.

In the Elimination Diet you will follow a plan that in the simplest sense removes all the irritating foods and adds in all the healing and nourishing foods. Performing this shift in what you eat every day will produce incredibly profound results. It can increase energy, drop weight, relieve pain, produce intestinal peace, and lift moods. And that's just the tip of the iceberg.

In our lifetimes, we are going to take close to 25 tons of foreign particles from the outside world into our mouths as food. This food will contain essential nutrients we need for health. But it will also contain bacteria, parasites, curiously shaped food proteins, and a host of compounds that could have a negative effect on our systems.

As a result, some of the foods you are eating currently are likely irritating your intestines (also known as your gut). As you will learn later in this book, when you irritate your intestines, you irritate your entire system. You have to create a calm gut before you can truly feel better. And to do this, you have to remove all the potential trigger foods—you'll learn all about these in chapter 3.

HOW YOU COULD BE OVERREACTING TO FOODS

Every time you take a bite of food, your body has a reaction. Many of these reactions are normal and essential—you need foods to signal the release of enzymes and other chemicals in order for the digestion process to take place. But there are other types of reactions that can occur that aren't so productive; in fact, they can be downright destructive.

We'll look at these reactions in two categories: food allergies and food intolerance. You've likely heard of food allergies or been affected by them personally. While they've historically been rare, they are becoming more common, especially among school-age children.

Food intolerance is less well known, but is a concept you're likely going to hear a lot about in the coming years. This latter reaction usually creates a subtler, simmering sort of distress that leads to chronic symptoms. Let's explore them both a bit further.

FOOD ALLERGY

All allergic responses are a result of something directly triggering the immune system. If you have a **food allergy**, your immune cells have recognized a particular portion of a food as harmful and have produced a specific antibody to combat that food. An antibody, otherwise known as an immunoglobulin, is a protein that will help neutralize an allergen directly or signal for help from the rest of the immune system. The antibody most commonly associated with allergies is known as an immunoglobulin E (IgE) antibody.

Once the body has identified a food allergen, the immune cells will produce IgE antibodies each time it's eaten. The antibodies will bind to the allergenic food and also to the immune cells in the local area, causing redness, swelling, heat, pain, and itching. Since the majority of your immune cells are in the gut, digestive issues may also accompany the reaction.

Allergic reactions can be immediate or develop within a few hours, and create symptoms such as:

- Swelling in the face, tongue, throat, and lips
- Wheezing and difficulty with breathing
- Red and itchy skin, often with hives
- Vomiting and/or diarrhea

When severe, these reactions may be life threatening.

Even though typical IgE allergenic reactions are only a small fraction of food reactions, they've increased over the last couple of decades. A 2013 study by the Centers for Disease Control (CDC) showed that food allergies have increased 50 percent from 1997 to 2011. According to a 2010 article in the *Journal of Allergy and Clinical Immunology*, there was a 300 percent rise in peanut allergies from 1997 to 2008. Over half the population of the United States tests positive to at least one allergen, yet few have pinpointed the source of their symptoms.

Ninety percent of all IgE food allergies in the United States can be attributed to 8 food groups: milk, eggs, fish, crustacean shellfish, wheat, soy, peanuts, and tree nuts. Many of these same foods also cause food reactions that are not IgE related, and these are much more common.

Beyond the typical IgE allergies, there are numerous other possible immune responses that could be triggered by foods. Your immune cells can produce other types of antibodies, such as IgG, IgM, and IgA. These are sometimes referred to as non-IgE-related food allergies or labeled as food "sensitivities."

While these types of reactions are not as well studied or understood as IgE reactions, they are a far more common cause of food-based reactions. And they are likely a hidden source of your symptoms. The key in all of these "allergic reactions" is that the food proteins are stimulating an immune cell response.

To test for IgE allergies, a doctor might suggest a skin-prick test and radioallergosorbent testing (RAST), but they're not guaranteed to identify the source of your symptoms. These tests are notorious for not being entirely accurate for IgE reactions, and they are not designed to pick up non-IgE reactions.

The tests that *are* designed for non-IgE food reactions are not always reliable for every person. In my clinical practice, I have seen IgG food panels or IgA oral food reaction tests miss some reactions while giving false positives on others. While helpful for picking up some sensitivity reactions that IgE testing will not, I do not consider the results from these tests definitive for food reactions.

The reality is that lab tests are imperfect; they are looking for a specific reaction to a specific protein in foods. Because there are thousands of chemicals in foods that you might react to, it's incredibly difficult to get accurate answers. The most reliable way to determine if you are having negative reactions to a food is to follow an elimination diet.

FOOD INTOLERANCE

A food intolerance is often a delayed and undetected food reaction. It does not directly involve the immune system secreting antibodies, but may cause the immune cells to get activated indirectly.

Intolerances are usually due to the body not being able to process a component of a particular food. For instance, one of the most common intolerances is lactose intolerance, which is present when a person lacks adequate amounts of the enzyme lactase. You need lactase, which is produced on the surface of your intestinal cells, to break down lactose, a sugar found in milk. Around 60 to 75 percent of the world's population doesn't have enough lactase after the age of 4 to adequately digest the lactose found in many milk products. As a result, many of those people will suffer from something called lactose intolerance.

When you can't process a type of food, it's an indication that you're lacking an enzyme, nutrient, or organism that's needed to properly digest or metabolize a substance. This means each time you eat this food, more of the undigested particles will build up in the body, feeding organisms that live in your intestinal tract, such as bacteria and yeast, and/or producing harmful effects.

Most people are intolerant to at least one food, and plenty others react poorly to multiple foods. Without knowing it, you might be intolerant to a food you're eating every day. *Have you ever stopped to consider what is behind your bloating, cramping, constipation, diarrhea, migraine, skin problems, or joint pain? Do they happen after you've eaten a certain food?* Many of these symptoms will present themselves shortly after you eat a food to which you're intolerant, or they might not be noticeable for a couple days.

How do you know if you have a food intolerance? Let's take a look at lactose intolerance again. If you are lactose intolerant, within 30 minutes to 2 hours after you eat dairy products that contain lactose (e.g., milk, ice cream, cheese), you might experience symptoms of gas, bloating, nausea, cramping, and diarrhea. These symptoms are a result of resident microbes taking over digestion because the body can't do it on its own. As these microbes eat/break down these milk sugars, they release gas that can cause you to bloat and feel miserable. If you've consumed lactose in high quantities, the body signals for a release of fluids to flush the undigested substance out of the intestines, which you'll experience as more bloating and cramping, and then later as diarrhea.

This is just one example of how a person's body may not tolerate a particular food. Intolerances to other food substances, such as amines found in fermented foods, phenols in food additives and berries, fructose from fruits and high-fructose corn syrup, and glutamate in MSG and high-protein foods, are gaining in prevalence.

Symptoms can be across the board for food intolerances:

- Foggy thinking
- Mood issues (anxiety, depression)
- Bowel problems (gas, nausea, bloating, cramping, diarrhea, constipation)
- Sinus and lung problems (asthma, sinusitis, otitis media, bronchitis, postnasal drip)
- Headaches

- Unexplained weight gain
- Low energy
- Insomnia
- Skin disorders
- Joint pain and muscle pain

Most lab tests do not test for food intolerances at all. People often come into my clinical practice with extensive lab results and say they are confused. Their tests say they should *not* be reacting to things like corn, soy, gluten, or sesame seeds, and yet they're experiencing rashes, headaches, or stomach distress shortly after consuming them. Even clients with celiac disease, an autoimmune disease triggered by an allergy to gluten, have tested negative on IgG food panels, despite their reactions to gluten being clear and severe.

Lab tests can even reveal a false positive, or an incorrect source of reaction. I once had several clients test positive for asparagus from a particular lab, which seemed suspicious. We later found out that there was an error in the testing process itself. After years of clinical experience, I always question lab results and assume there is a margin for error. That's why I always recommend the Elimination Diet as step one.

THE GUT–BRAIN CONNECTION

Have you ever eaten something and then gotten a headache? Or found that a meal left you feeling anxious? What you feel in your head can sometimes begin in the gut. Nerve endings in the intestinal lining lead directly to the brain; this connection allows for food particles, bacteria, or chemicals in the intestines to cause a change in behavior and mood. People who have trouble breaking down food substances like amines and glutamates (think monosodium glutamate, commonly known as MSG) might also experience side effects when these build up in the body. Amines can constrict blood vessels and lead to headaches, while glutamates can overexcite the brain, leading to feelings of anxiety.

THE TWISTED, UNHEALTHY RELATIONSHIP OF FOOD INTOLERANCE AND INFLAMMATION

You might be having a food reaction every day, or multiple times a day, without even knowing it. Your symptoms might be mild, moderate, or severe, and your motivation to determine the source of your symptoms probably varies accordingly.

By the time they come to me, many of my clients are nearly hopeless and often in a great deal of discomfort—they will try anything to experience relief. If you aren't there yet, be thankful. But you should know that there's danger in letting more subtle symptoms pass by undetected and untreated. They are a sign of a slow-burning fire inside that's quietly (or not so quietly) and chronically causing damage and irritation to your cells. This steady fire is what's known as inflammation.

Inflammation is part of your body's immune response to anything flagged as harmful or irritating. You want it to occur when you bang your shin on the coffee table, because inflammatory proteins will help tissues heal and repair. You don't want it to occur in a chronic state.

When chronic low-grade inflammation is present, even harmless substances like food particles, beneficial bacteria, and the cells of your own tissues are likely to become targets. It is not normal for your body to attack the cells of your thyroid gland (Hashimoto's thyroiditis), your pancreas (type 1 diabetes), or your joints (rheumatoid arthritis). And these are just a few of the conditions associated with chronic inflammation. Inflammatory chemicals can also lead to plaque buildup in the arteries (atherosclerosis), high blood pressure, sleep apnea, and even depression.

A 2008 study published in *Experimental Clinical Endocrinology and Diabetes* explored the connection between food reactions and inflammation. Researchers discovered that overweight children were two and a half times more likely to have reactions to foods than their normal-weight counterparts. They also had increased levels of inflammation, instigated by food reactions, and three times greater arterial wall thickening, a precursor to heart disease. The authors summarized their findings by stating that immune reactions to food are likely "involved in the development of obesity and atherosclerosis."

Food intolerance and inflammation have an intimate and complicated relationship—they can each bring about the other. When you have undetected and unresolved food intolerance, the irritation will fester and grow to the point of creating chronic inflammation. On the flip side, if inflammation is present due to other irritants, such as environmental toxins and processed foods, you can be more prone to developing food intolerance.

In either case, your immune system and intestinal tract are hotbeds of distress. When inflammation is ongoing, there will be a continuous presence of inflammatory chemicals. When this happens in the gut—where 70 percent of the immune cells reside—it can create damage to the intestinal barrier and lead to leaky gut, a condition you'll read more about on page 44.

THE OTHER INFLAMMATORY TRIGGERS IN YOUR LIFE

Inflammation happens every time your immune system has to fend off irritants that come into the body, and poorly tolerated food particles aren't the only common irritants we encounter.

Some of the other everyday irritants that trigger an inflammatory response are:

- Bad bacteria in our food, water, and air
- Environmental toxins (pesticides, PCBs, and dioxins)
- Non-food-based allergens (dust mites, pollen, dander)
- Processed foods (sugar, trans fats, food additives)
- Stress

Our current rate of exposure to many of these triggers is off the charts (I'll go into more detail about this in chapter 4). The average American consumes 152 pounds of sugar a year and is exposed constantly to more than 10,000 chemicals used as additives in the food supply. More than 74 *billion* pounds of chemicals are being produced in or imported into the United

States every single day—that number doesn't even include pesticides, food additives, fuels, or pharmaceuticals.

The odds are high that if you're living in modern society, you endure daily insults to your immune system that can create an enduring inflamed state. Whether you are aware of it or not, your body is responding. It speaks in symptoms, which are the body's way of saying that something is out of balance. To quiet the symptoms, you must remove the irritants. With the Elimination Diet, we start with the most likely source: food.

HOW THE ELIMINATION DIET WORKS

With the Elimination Diet, our goal is to use food to calm inflammation and restore balance to the body. We accomplish this with a three-phase plan, which has been improved and updated over the years based on client results and additional research. The first phase is a detoxification phase (Detox), the second will feature balancing neutral foods (Elimination), and the third and final phase will be when you add back potentially reactive foods (Reintroduction). Here's a little more on each phase:

Detox: The Detoxification Phase will begin to calm the immune system and clear the gut. This phase consists only of fresh vegetable juices, green smoothies, and puréed cooked vegetables in bone broth.

Elimination: The Elimination Phase is a baseline diet, consisting of anti-inflammatory foods that normally don't cause an immune response in most people.

During this phase, you'll remove processed and potentially irritating foods from your diet. Through ten years of clinical experience, and reviews of hundreds of research articles, I have put together a specific list of foods that are more likely than others to irritate your body. Gluten and dairy have repeatedly proven to be among the most damaging and irritating substances. But we'll also remove the other trigger foods, including:

- Eggs
- Yeast
- Corn
- Sugar
- Citrus

- Coffee
- Chocolate
- Beef
- Pork
- Tree nuts
- Peanuts

To replace those foods, you'll be filling your plate with foods full of beneficial chemicals and calming compounds. These foods will help repair your damaged cells and heal your gut.

Reintroduction: This is where foods are added back in, one by one, to see if you are having a reaction. A diet diary will be especially important during this phase as we identify your distinct food responses. Once your gas, nausea, bloating, skin problems, pain, headaches, or fatigue go away, you can add potentially irritating foods back in one at a time to see which ones trigger your symptoms. Once you know, you will have found the optimal diet program for your unique body and can experience an entirely new level of health.

CALORIES DON'T COUNT

The best part of the Elimination Diet is there is absolutely no focus on calories. You are eating for energy, healing, and pristine metabolic function—you can eat often and as much as you want of organic, whole, anti-inflammatory foods. The extensive food lists and hundreds of recipes offered in this book will ensure you have plenty of options with which to fill your plate!

The vast majority of people who enter the doors of my office, or consult with me over the phone, get significantly better when following this Elimination Diet. Many have life-altering experiences.

THE CUSTOMIZED DIET EXPERIENCE

There's a reason the Elimination Diet is so powerful and should be the first step you take toward stopping your symptoms: It offers the ultimate in diet customization. You may have tried other diets without success, but none of them were built to improve your unique system.

Even if you have a hunch of what's contributing to your weight gain, joint pain, or irritable bowel symptoms, you won't find a better way to test it than the Elimination Diet. The best way to figure out what works best for your system is to take out the primary irritants and see how you feel.

2

THE GLORIOUS GUT

This chapter will teach you how to evaluate your own digestion and figure out what your gut is trying to tell you: You will learn to listen to your (literal) gut. Gaining a basic understanding of the digestion process will be a big asset to you as you begin to connect the dots between the foods you eat and your unwanted symptoms.

When normal digestion is taking place, you are absorbing life-giving nutrients from food; your body's natural immunity is at its strongest; and waste and toxins are properly filtered out of the body. It's a perfect system. But when things go wrong here, things can go wrong everywhere.

Digestion, the process of breaking your food from large pieces to small pieces, will allow you to access all the nutrition stored in the food you eat. It takes place primarily in your mouth with chewing and enzymes in your saliva, your stomach with stomach acid, and your upper intestines with bile from your gallbladder, digestive enzymes from your pancreas, and digestive enzymes from the lining of your intestines.

When you are having reactions to foods, these very same areas where digestion is taking place can become inflamed and dysfunctional. This can slow down and interfere with the process of digestion of your food. Undigested food is food that cannot pass into your body in the form of nutrients. If you can't access the nutrients from your food, your body will begin to function differently. Processes important to metabolism, energy, and cell and tissue health, to name just a few, will stall and not function properly. You will also have to process this extra waste of undigested food that is now sitting in your intestinal tract. This clearing of waste is often what causes the unwanted symptoms of gas, nausea, bloating, diarrhea, and/or constipation.

Seventy million people in the world are plagued by symptoms like these, and if you're reading this book, my guess is that you are, too. The good news is that these symptoms and more will get better with the Elimination Diet. To better understand your symptoms and what's causing them, let's take a tour of the digestive processes that take place in the gut.

THE WHOLE GUT STORY

So, what is the gut? Otherwise known as the gastrointestinal (GI) tract, your gut is the long and winding tube that begins at the mouth and ends at the anus. *Science* magazine named it "the inner tube of life," which couldn't be more appropriate—without the gut, we could not feed the cells of the body and keep critical systems up and running.

Digestion, or the breaking down of food, occurs within this inner tube, which is sealed off from the other parts of the body. That's because food particles and the enzymes and acids required for the processing of these particles would be useless at best and toxic at worst if they were to make their way into other areas of the body (more on this when we get to the trouble with a leaky gut on page 44).

When you eat, food should be transported through the body in this order: mouth, esophagus, stomach, small intestines, large intestines. Each part is responsible for a distinct and important role in this awesome assembly line, from the initial breakdown of foods to the final elimination of waste. The system is anything but a garbage disposal composed of molecules; the gut is a highly intelligent and efficient epicenter of communication, nutrient management, and immune function.

Digestion in its entirety can take up to 40 hours, depending on meal composition—proteins, carbs, fat, and fiber are all broken down differently—and your individual digestive health. Here's a little more on what happens when you eat a piece of food.

IN THE MOUTH

It all begins even before food hits your mouth, when you see and smell the food and your body begins to prep itself for digestion. Once food enters your mouth, your teeth will perform most of the hard labor as bites of food are broken down into smaller pieces.

GET TOOTHY WITH IT

In 2009, a group of researchers with the Department of Foods and Nutrition at Purdue University tested the number of chews of a food and its impact on nutrient absorption. They wanted to know if the amount of times an almond was chewed would affect how much of it was absorbed into the body and used for energy. They compared people chewing 10, 25, or 40 times before swallowing. The results, published in the *American Journal of Clinical Nutrition*, were clear: the more chews (40), the greater the energy extracted for use. Fewer chews (10 or 25) led to more of the nutrients from almonds being discarded as toilet trash. Don't waste energy—chew your food!

Little proteins called enzymes will assist the chewing process in the breakdown of foods. These enzymes, many of which are recognizable by the suffix "–ase," are brilliant at changing the shape of hundreds of thousands of things. Our food is a prime example. We use enzymes from our mouths to break apart carbohydrates (salivary amylase) and give a little boost to fat digestion later on in the stomach (salivary lipase).

What Can Go Wrong Here

Food particles that aren't completely broken down in the mouth can lead later to gas, nausea, bloating, diarrhea, or constipation. You'll also risk missing out on valuable nutrition if you don't let your teeth do their job well. Slow down and savor your food and you'll do your digestion and the rest of your body a big favor.

IN THE STOMACH

When the food drops down from the esophagus into the stomach, it will fall into a pool of gastric acid. This acid breaks apart food and destroys harmful bacteria, viruses, and parasites. You want strong stomach acid! The pH level of the acid in the stomach of a healthy person is very similar to that of battery acid (around 1.7). If you dropped your food into battery acid, you would see it disintegrate over a relatively short period of time (don't try this at home). The same thing happens in your stomach.

The acidic breakdown is essential for you to access all the vitamins, minerals, proteins, and other nutrients "trapped" in foods. Acid also helps the body absorb certain foods. Important nutrients like vitamin B12, iron, folates (formerly known as folic acid), and zinc are all absorbed better in an acid-rich environment. Without the acid, nutrient deficiencies are far more common.

When your foods are properly digested by stomach acid, your stomach is calm after you eat. There is less of a chance for bloating, gas, belching, and reflux.

What Can Go Wrong Here

The term *indigestion* literally means a lack of digestion. Many people assume when they have indigestion, it's because they have too much acid in their stomach. To feel better, they might take medications like Prilosec, Prevacid, Pepcid, and Zantac, which turn off the ability to produce acid. Medical doctors will prescribe acid-blocking medications based on a similar assumption that the majority of cases of GERD, bloating, stomach pain, or indigestion are due to high acid levels in the stomach.

The problem is, what's really going on with a lot of people is not too much stomach acid, but too little. In fact, research indicates that only a third of the prescriptions of acid-blocking medications are warranted. When my friend and colleague Dr. Adam Geiger tested for stomach acid on several patients, he found high stomach acid to be a practically nonexistent condition. Using a Heidelberg test that measures stomach acid function, he tested 199 consecutive patients varying from 7 to 86 years old (average age of 54) who had come to see him with indigestion, bloating, diarrhea, reflux, constipation, and other issues.

Out of the 199 patients tested, 0 percent had too much stomach acid. Zero. Only 21 percent had normal levels of stomach acid, while the remaining 79 percent had varying degrees of insufficient stomach acid secretion. A surprising 22 percent were severely deficient. While these are unpublished results, it is quite possible that people are receiving prescriptions for medications that are counterproductive.

In fact, long-term or heavy use of acid-blocking medications has some potentially serious side effects. They can weaken your stomach acid so much that it has the effectiveness of table vinegar, literally: According to an article in the *Journal of Gastroenterology*, the average pH of a person taking a common acid-blocking therapy (omeprazole) will be similar to that of table vinegar (pH of 5) within five days of taking the medication.

In this state, you're at risk for nutrient deficiencies and bacterial infections. Research, including work published by Dr. Joel J. Heidelbaugh in the *American Journal of Gastroenterology*, has identified risks between these meds and diminished levels of the essential bone minerals calcium and magnesium, and the essential brain nutrient B12. They've also been connected to increased risk of infection from a bacterium by the name of *Clostridium difficile*, a nasty, diarrhea-causing bug.

Decreased stomach acid creates an environment ineffective at food breakdown. If your foods are not properly broken down, your immune system may mistake the larger food fragments for foreign invaders and launch an attack. In 2005, a group of researchers in Vienna led by Dr. Eva Untersmayr discovered that subjects who were lowering stomach acid with medication had a 300 percent increase in allergenic IgE antibodies, were 10.5 times more likely to develop food-specific allergies, and had a significant increase in airborne allergies as well.

TEST YOUR STOMACH ACID

This simple test is highly recommended if you have bloating or mineral deficiencies of calcium and magnesium. You can test your own gastric acid function using the betaine HCL challenge, a method that has been used for many decades by alternative medicine practitioners.

The idea of this test is to put more acid in your system and see how it affects your symptoms. If your symptoms improve with supplemental acid, it can be assumed that you may be low in stomach acid and need to supplement on a regular basis to enhance normal digestion.

The test is suggested if you're experiencing symptoms such as gas, nausea, bloating, GERD, diarrhea, or constipation. It is not recommended for people who are currently taking gastric acid blocking medications, or have a recent history of ulcers or use of corticosteroids (prednisone) and non-steroidal anti-inflammatory drugs (NSAIDs) like aspirin, ibuprofen

(Advil, Motrin), naproxin (Aleve), and COX-2 inhibitors (Celebrex). These substances together with betaine HCL can damage stomach and intestinal tissues.

To perform the test, pick up betaine HCL with pepsin, which you can find at most supplement stores. Look for a high-quality variety, ideally with no lactose, stearates (magnesium stearate, stearic acid), or palmitates (palmitic acid, ascrobyl palmitate).

After the first few bites of your next meal containing protein, take one capsule. Finish your meal and journal what happens with your symptoms. You are looking for a warming sensation in your stomach, an increase in appetite, or a lessening of bloating, nausea, gas, and diarrhea. If you experienced any of these after just one capsule, you likely have sufficient stomach acid.

If you didn't feel a warming sensation, continue to take one capsule per meal for one full day. If, at any time, you get a cramping or burning sensation, stop taking the betaine HCL. Drinking a glass of water with a teaspoon of baking soda in it or eating more food will quickly ease any cramping or burning.

If you do not notice any symptom changes at all, start taking 2 capsules per meal the next day. Continue adding in one cap per day until you notice that warming or a change in your symptoms. Most people find this occurs between 4 and 7 capsules per meal.

To manage low gastric acid, once you have found the number of capsules that changes your symptoms back that number down by one. If you noticed an increase of appetite and a warming of your stomach at 5 capsules, start taking 4 caps with every major meal. Stay with this amount until you notice those symptoms again. Over time you may need to back down one more capsule per meal.

Be conscious of the fact that small meals, or meals low in protein, may need less, and those with more protein, or harder to digest foods (like nuts and seeds, or steak), may need more.

If you experience acid reflux and heartburn, it's highly likely that food is creating your discomfort, not an excess of gastric acid. Food reactions to things like gluten, dairy, caffeine, citrus, alcohol, and nightshade vegetables can all trigger acid reflux. So, too, can being overweight and having a hiatal hernia. The power of the Elimination Diet is that it will reveal to you the true source of your discomfort and (ideally) free you from the need to take unnecessary medications with superfluous side effects.

IN THE SMALL INTESTINES

In the small intestines, you have three important players of the digestive process: the intestinal cells themselves, the bile from the gallbladder, and the enzymes that get secreted from the pancreas. As our food passes into the upper intestinal region, the cells there will release a hormone called cholecystokinin (CCK), which will in turn signal the gallbladder to secrete bile and the pancreas to secrete digestive enzymes. These substances are essential to helping you get the most nutrients from foods.

Since these cells and organs serve separate but complementary functions, let's get to know them on an individual basis.

The Intestinal Cells

The cells that line the intestinal wall act like "bookends" of the digestion process that occurs within the small intestines. In the beginning, they excrete CCK to trigger the release of bile and digestive enzymes. And at the end, they will secrete "brush border" enzymes that take the final pieces of carbohydrates and proteins and break them into single sugars and amino acids, respectively, which the body can then absorb.

What Can Go Wrong Here

When damage has occurred to the cells and CCK and enzyme production has been disturbed, digestive distress and a leaky gut (see page 44 for more on leaky gut) can begin to develop.

The problem is that we're consistently exposed to elements that upset intestinal cells. Toxins, unfriendly inhabitants of the intestines (parasites, viruses, bacteria, yeasts), medications (aspirin, naproxen, ibuprofen), and psychological stress can irritate and inflame these important cells. But by far the most irritating substance of all is food. Alcohol, dairy, soy, and high-fructose corn syrup can aggravate intestinal cells, but wheat is the worst. A 2004 article in the journal *Pancreas* showed that lectins—proteins that bind to carbohydrates—in wheat, called wheat germ agglutinin, are capable of limiting CCK secretion by as much as 70 percent.

TEST YOUR CCK LEVELS

If CCK levels are low, fats will not be properly digested and absorbed. This can lead to cramping, bloating, diarrhea, and urgent bowel movements. You can do a simple at-home test to see if you're producing enough CCK:

- Take one tablespoon of purified fish oil twice a day, morning and night.
- Monitor your digestive reaction. If your stools are lighter colored and floating, you produce foul-smelling gas, and/or you experience urgent bowel movements, your CCK secretion is likely low.

If you do find this is an issue, taking a pancreatic enzyme supplement with ox bile or conjugated bile acids will likely be helpful in lessening your symptoms. Consult a skilled Functional Medicine practitioner for proper diagnosis and treatment of these issues. (For more information, see the information on digestive enzymes in Supplements to Support the Elimination Diet on page 107.)

The Gallbladder

The gallbladder secretes bile to process fats found in foods. It works a bit like dish detergent does on greasy, fatty food remnants by splitting them apart or emulsifying them. Have you ever seen dish detergent break down fats that have floated to the top of a sink full of water? The soap will literally break apart all of the fat globules into small beadlets; this is exactly what bile does with the fats in your food.

Another important function of bile is to clear out excessive toxins from your liver. The liver is the body's primary filter for toxins. Once the liver has done its job of processing toxins, they'll get disposed of by way of bile.

What Can Go Wrong Here

If the gallbladder is slow to release bile or doesn't produce enough of it (due to insufficient CCK), a few troubling things can occur. First, fats might not get processed into small enough pieces to get absorbed into your body. These unabsorbed fats can wreak havoc by forming substances that literally "wash" out your intestines, causing looser and floating stools.

Second, if the gallbladder doesn't regularly release bile, it can build up within the organ and cause gallbladder stasis, or stuck bile, which can lead to gallstones. Gallbladder disease can also develop.

And third, an absence of enough bile will allow for toxins to build up within the body.

Food reactions, primarily to gluten, have been shown to slow the release of bile and to decrease overall gallbladder function. Reactions can create problems by causing inflammation in the intestinal cells. When these cells are irritated, less CCK is produced, which you'll remember you need to trigger the release of bile from the gallbladder.

Gallbladder diseases have been associated with food sensitivities since the 1940s, but very few people have paid any attention to the medical records of that era. In 1968, Dr. Brenemen published an article in the *Annals of Allergy* entitled "Allergy elimination diet as the most effective gallbladder diet," where he found strong links between foods and gallbladder dysfunction. You can see some foods like eggs, pork, and onions caused a reaction in more than half of the people with gallbladder issues:

Food	Percentage of patients reacting
Eggs	93%
Pork	64%
Onions	52%
Fowl	35%
Milk	25%
Coffee	22%
Oranges	19%
Corn	15%
Beans	15%
Nuts	15%
Apples	6%
Tomatoes	6%

CASE STUDY

Jody was a celiac client who had no outward symptoms at all. She found out that she had celiac disease after being diagnosed with a chronic iron deficiency. She had been supplementing with iron for years and yet it wasn't being properly absorbed. Jody was finally sent to a gastroenterologist to get her upper intestinal tract checked, since this is where most of the iron should be absorbed. It turns out her intestinal tract was worn down by years of eating gluten. She was diagnosed as having celiac disease and was told the genes were passed on to her by her parents.

Late one night, I received a phone call from Jody that sounded rather urgent. She was quite excited and out of breath when she asked: "Tom, have you read any research saying that gallbladder function can be associated with celiac disease?" I replied yes, and she quickly hung up the phone.

A few days later, I received a phone call from her thanking me profusely. Her mother, Marge, had been suffering from gallbladder attacks for many years, and she had just recently canceled a trip to Australia days before she was to leave due to an attack.

When I received the call from Jody, Marge was having a terrible attack that brought her to the emergency room. Marge was about to have her gallbladder removed when, for some reason, Jody got a strong feeling that celiac disease was behind the attacks. She pleaded with the doctors to test Marge for celiac disease before doing surgery, and they agreed.

They confirmed that she had celiac disease. She got to keep her gallbladder, but she was going to have to drop gluten from her diet. Marge now lives a life free of suffering and full of quilt making. She delivered to me gifts of gratitude for each of my children: the most beautiful fleece-lined quilts that you have ever seen. Now, as I tuck my kids in at night, I am constantly reminded of the power food has on the gallbladder.

The Pancreas

Enzymes that are released by the pancreas are key to the digestion of proteins, carbs, and fats.

What Can Go Wrong Here

Without proper enzyme function, food particles are left to be digested by organisms that live in the intestinal tract, such as bacteria and yeast. Feeding certain strains of bacteria and yeast can lead to bacterial and fungal imbalances that are associated with irritable bowel and a host of other diseases and disorders.

It's possible to look to your bowel movements to see if you have enough digestive enzymes (yes, I'm talking about poop). If your bowel movements float; are lighter orange, gray, or brown; are urgent, foul smelling, and often looser, this is an indication that you aren't digesting fats very well and could have a condition call steatorrhea. In this case, along with the ox bile and bile acids mentioned earlier, you could benefit from taking digestive enzymes, particularly those high in lipases, which are dedicated to digesting fats.

If you see lots of undigested food particles in your stool, but know you chewed well when eating your meals, this is an indication that your digestive enzymes are not working.

My clients with irritated bowels have found that they feel better when taking digestive enzymes. Research in 2007 by Leeds et al. has shown that a digestive enzyme supplement can effectively reduce the frequency of loose stools in people suffering from multiple loose bowel movements a day (from 4 or more down to 1). The removal of dairy and gluten from the diet can also be effective at improving enzyme production, by way of promoting healthy CCK secretion.

IN THE LARGE INTESTINES

The large intestines, which include the colon, play a large indirect role in digestion. It's here that the highest concentration of bacteria and other beneficial organisms reside. (For more on these beneficial bacteria, see Your Bacterial Best Friends on page 41.) Up to 50 percent of your daily folate (B9) needs could be coming from the bacteria in your colon. But they don't stop there. The bacterial flora in the colon also manufacture and supply tryptophan, phenylalanine, tyrosine, riboflavin (B2), niacin (B3), pantothenic acid (B5), pyridoxine (B6), biotin (B7), and vitamin K2.

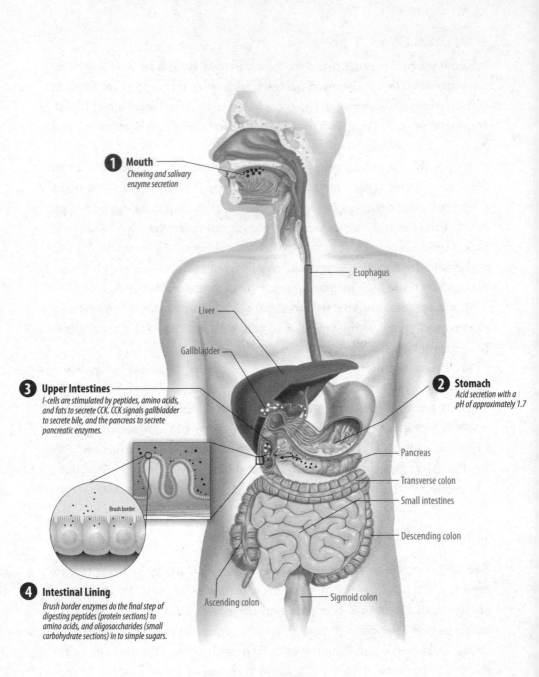

1 **Mouth**
Chewing and salivary enzyme secretion

Esophagus

Liver

Gallbladder

3 **Upper Intestines**
I-cells are stimulated by peptides, amino acids, and fats to secrete CCK. CCK signals gallbladder to secrete bile, and the pancreas to secrete pancreatic enzymes.

Brush border

4 **Intestinal Lining**
Brush border enzymes do the final step of digesting peptides (protein sections) to amino acids, and oligosaccharides (small carbohydrate sections) in to simple sugars.

2 **Stomach**
Acid secretion with a pH of approximately 1.7

Pancreas

Transverse colon

Small intestines

Descending colon

Ascending colon

Sigmoid colon

The Digestive System

YOUR BACTERIAL BEST FRIENDS

It's clear the gut is essential to processing the food you eat and making it usable for the body. But that's really only part of the big picture when it comes to the glorious gut. You might remember we have a rich and populated bacterial ecosystem within the gut, called the gut microbiome. This bacterial haven holds over 100 trillion microorganisms that are exposed to whatever enters your mouth: food, particles, toxins, hair stubble, bugs... you name it.

In the healthy gut, most of the bacteria are commensal; that is, they're ready and willing to help you fend off pathogens and remove toxins as long as you keep the living conditions up to their standards. They don't ask for much: Nutrient-rich foods with plenty of plant fibers, a calm and peaceful state, and an absence of excessive chemicals are just a few of their favorite things.

When we have a diverse and plentiful microbiome, the intestinal cells keep the digestive process running smoothly and the immune system calm. The cells actually take roll call on what microorganisms are present. When they can check off plenty of good guys in attendance, they send a message to the immune system signifying that all is well.

Once the immune system gets the message, it knows to stay calm and let food and healthy cells pass by. It's only when beneficial bacteria begin to disappear that the intestinal and immune cells will flare up into a state of alarm, increasing inflammation and digestive irritation.

Disappearances of beneficial bacteria have been linked to a greater risk for insulin resistance, type 2 diabetes, chronic inflammation, and increased weight gain.

It's possible that you might be unintentionally squelching your good bacteria. Here are some factors that can push out beneficial bacteria and make room for the bad:

- Antibiotics, anti-inflammatories, and other common medications
- Chronic stress (physical and emotional)
- Diet high in processed and pesticide-laden foods
- Exposure to toxins
- Excessive use of antibacterial products
- Low stomach acid (which lets pathogenic bacteria run wild)

The upside is that while the gut microbiome is sensitive, it's also highly responsive. A 2014 study published in the journal *Nature* revealed that a change in your diet can create rapid shifts in the bacterial environment. Researchers fed various diets to subjects and they followed their changes of microbes in their intestinal tract. Surprisingly, it only took three days before significant shifts took place. This means when you follow the Elimination Diet, you can produce profound changes in your body quickly by eating the kinds of foods that help the beneficial bacteria thrive and kill off the bad bacteria. Restoring balance to your microbiome will lead to greater relief from symptoms, especially those related to GI distress.

To help restore and replenish your beneficial bacteria during the Elimination Diet, you should:

- Get more probiotics and prebiotics
- Eliminate the most common food irritants: gluten, dairy, egg, corn, soy, yeast
- Eat plenty of fermented foods like sauerkraut, dosas, coconut kefir, and lacto-fermented veggies

Throughout the book, you'll find information and guidance on how to do each of these things.

THE GREAT GUT BARRIER

It's hard to believe it, but all the food particles, enzymes, gastric acid, and over 100-trillion-strong bacterial ecosystem fit within the inner tube of the gut.

The contents of the GI tract are so strictly cordoned off from the other areas of the body that they're *separate from the rest of* the body. Let's think about this for a second. We have a tube that runs through our body and a large portion of the contents of this tube is *never* intended to actually pass into our bodies. Things like bacteria and undigested food particles are supposed to be kept in this tube. So, what's responsible for keeping track of what stays out and what goes in? The intestinal barrier.

The intestinal barrier, or lining of the gut, is a layer of single cells all tightly stuck together by a number of compounds. When these cells form tight junctions, you have an incredibly dynamic barrier that protects your insides from the contents of your intestines.

But the barrier isn't just an inert protector. On the outside of the wall, the intestinal cells are busy secreting substances like mucus, IgA antibodies, and little antimicrobial peptides that all protect the gut from harm and keep pathogens in check.

Your intestinal cells need to be healthy and strong to maintain this multifunctional barrier. And yet today, it's more common for them to be surrounded by damaging substances rather than nourishing ones. These cells are harmed by:

- Harmful bacteria
- Medications
- Reactive foods
- Rough food (think sharp corn chips) or fibrous substances
- Toxins

Basically, once in the intestines, these substances will cause damage to the intestinal lining. By design, the cells are resilient and constantly rebuilding themselves to fortify the barrier. In fact, your intestinal cells are replicating so fast that your entire small intestines will have new cells every three days. But this constant replacement takes a ton of energy and nutrients like B vitamins, amino acids, and zinc. If you're eating a diet high in nutrient-rich, calming foods, your intestinal cells can recover and repair quickly. If instead you're eating gut-irritating, cell-inflaming foods or nutrient-depleted foods, the stage is set for a cascade into a full-blown inflammatory state.

Having inflamed, damaged cells within the intestines is asking for trouble. Chemicals will be secreted to heal the damaged tissue. Those chemicals are supposed to create an environment where a posse of cells can rush in and repair the damage. Then they should disperse. When they don't—because the source of irritation is constant—the high concentration of chemicals will create unwanted damage in intestinal cells. Eventually, the chronic inflammatory response will lead to cracks in that critical barrier.

And then you have what's referred to as leaky gut syndrome.

LEAKY GUT SYNDROME

Leaky gut syndrome (LGS), also known as intestinal permeability, is a condition that natural health practitioners have been aware of and have been treating for years. It's finally gaining validation in the mainstream medical field, where associations between LGS and conditions such as type 2 diabetes, obesity, and autoimmune diseases like type 1 diabetes, celiac disease, and rheumatoid arthritis are being made.

When the bonds between the intestinal cells weaken, gaps in the barrier form and allow toxic chemicals and pathogenic viruses, parasites, and bacteria to sneak into the body. Your immune cells go nuts, working to combat the foreign invaders. Unfortunately, they use chemicals that cause collateral damage to the nearby intestinal lining.

In the midst of this chaos, the body works to maintain the energy and resources needed to metabolize food, produce energy, lubricate cells, utilize nutrients...and all the thousands of other jobs it has. But it can only do so much when there's a constant battle going on; eventually, something's got to give, and all too often it's your overall health that begins to suffer. Symptoms of leaky gut can include memory loss, brain fog, heavy fatigue, headaches, joint pain, skin rashes, chronic diarrhea or constipation...the sort of discomfort you wouldn't wish on your worst enemy.

The development of a leaky gut is often due to a variety of irritants to the intestines, but one stands out among the rest. The key culprit is something we bring into the body 3, 5, or 7 times a day: food.

Wheat and gluten are especially known to irritate the gut. That's because the carbohydrate-binding proteins in wheat (lectins) decrease the secretion of CCK, and the gliadin portion of gluten stimulates the release of a protein (zonulin) that leads to small permeations in even the most robust gut lining. (This means everyone is susceptible.)

While foods are the biggest category of irritants, they aren't the only factor to consider. These, in addition to gluten, are the most common things that contribute to a leaky gut:

- Acid-blocking medication
- Alcohol consumption
- Antibiotic use

- Environmental toxins—PCBs, mercury, pesticides, and others
- Excessive consumption of animal fats
- High fructose intake—from high-fructose corn syrup and agave nectar
- Immune-suppressing medication—corticosteroids, methotrexate
- Infections—bacteria (small intestinal bacterial overgrowth or SIBO), viral, parasitic, yeast
- Stress, or elevated cortisol levels (cortisol is a hormone released when you are under stress)
- Use of NSAIDs or non-steroid anti-inflammatories like aspirin, ibuprofen, and naproxen

The tricky thing about leaky gut is it can also create or worsen food sensitivities or intolerance. When the gut becomes permeable, you allow undigested components of food to sneak through. These unrecognized invaders are treated as dangerous compounds by the immune cells, and those cells launch an attack against the perceived invasion.

The immune system isn't one to easily forget the face of an invader; it's smart and proactive. It may form antibodies to be stored in its memory for future protection. Whenever you eat that food again, your immune cells attack. If you then eat that food 3 to 5 times a day, and you have a leaky gut, you will be in a constant state of alert and alarm with inflammatory chemicals circulating throughout your body.

AUTOIMMUNE DISEASE

Sometimes the immune system gets confused and our immune cells will start attacking a part of our own body. If it attacks the thyroid gland or thyroid-associated proteins, we end up with Hashimoto's thyroiditis. If it attacks the myelin sheath of our nerve cells, we can end up with multiple sclerosis. If it attacks the villi of our small intestines, we end up with celiac disease. This type of immune attack on the self is called an autoimmune disease.

Autoimmune diseases occur within an environment that is ripe for them. Dr. Alessio Fasano, a gastroenterologist with Massachusetts General Hospital in Boston and a world-renowned expert on celiac disease, noted in a study published in *Clinical Reviews in Allergy and Immunology* that there are 3 factors that leave a person susceptible to autoimmune disease:

1. Genetic predisposition
2. Exposure to environmental triggers or proteins that provoke an abnormal immune response
3. A leaky or permeable gut that allows these triggers to access the body

Since you can't change your genetics, the keys to reversing or preventing autoimmune disease will be healing your leaky gut and decreasing the exposure to food and bacterial proteins. Autoimmune diseases are more likely to develop if a person has had a leaky gut for a long time and has been eating foods that have been irritating it. This leads to a fragile environment of excessive inflammation and nutrient depletion.

The Elimination Diet will help both heal your leaky gut and reduce your exposure to food and bacterial proteins by:

1. eliminating the foods that are causing you harm
2. helping to build up a healthier balance of gut bacteria
3. supplementing with immune-boosting supplements such as vitamins A, D, K2, zinc, and essential fatty acids.

By following the program in this book, many people drastically reduce their symptoms, whether they are suffering from lupus, MS, rheumatoid arthritis, or Hashimoto's thyroiditis.

MAKING THE GUT WHOLE AGAIN

The amazing thing about the body is it wants to work perfectly, and it's extremely responsive to healing, enriching, replenishing nourishment. When a client presents symptoms of low stomach acid, insufficient digestive enzymes, and a leaky gut, I know the clearest course of action is the Elimination Diet. When we remove the primary irritants, we create the opportunity for bonds to reform in the intestinal barrier and for cells to regenerate. It's like giving your glorious gut a brand new start.

If you can start consuming antioxidant-rich vegetables, you can repair your gut. If you can start consuming meats that are lower in herbicides, pesticides, and mercury, you're not going to be irritated after you eat. You don't have to have headaches. You don't have to have bloating, gas, constipation, or an inflamed system planting the seeds of disease. You can heal your gut and be free of your symptoms by following the Elimination Diet. It all begins when we remove the primary irritants from your plate.

3

THE FOODS BEHIND YOUR SYMPTOMS

If you're like many of my patients, then you're probably all too familiar with uncomfortable symptoms like fatigue, bloating, heartburn, joint pain, and sinus issues.

Perhaps you've even been told before by doctors and other health-care professionals that there's nothing to be done about it. If that's the case, this chapter will be very exciting for you.

Part of our approach with the Elimination Diet is to treat your symptoms and your diet like a puzzle; you are a unique individual and there is a unique diet that will work best for you. This chapter is the first step toward piecing together your individualized diet. We start with an overview of the foods that are the most common culprits and the most frequent sources of symptoms. These are the most reactive foods and the foods most likely to cause intolerance. This doesn't mean that you'll necessarily have a reaction to all of these foods. But in order to pinpoint the diet that works best for you, we've got to remove these foods before you can experience freedom from your symptoms.

All the foods that appear in this chapter have the potential to damage and irritate the gut. When this irritation is persistent, leaky gut and chronic inflammation can develop, opening the door for autoimmune diseases and inflammatory conditions. We must focus first on removing these foods in order to create a calm and balanced environment within the gut.

In Part 3 of the book, you'll learn how to strategically remove and reintroduce these foods, which will enable you to create a customized diet. Here, I'd like to introduce you to them and their most irritating properties. My hope is that this will help you understand why they're being removed in the first place, and motivate you to stay on track throughout the program.

GLUTEN AND DAIRY: THE PRIMARY CULPRITS

More than 80 percent of my clients feel much better after eliminating gluten and dairy alone. Removing these two foods produces profound relief from such a wide array of symptoms that I often wonder why every single health-care practitioner doesn't begin treatment with this step.

Gluten

You've no doubt seen "gluten-free" foods start to take up more space at your grocery store, or gluten-free meals pop up on restaurant menus. Is this just a trend, driven by the latest fad diet? No, it's quite the opposite: It's a reflection of the market finally meeting the needs of the millions of people affected by gluten sensitivity. Whether you know it or not, you are likely one of those people.

Gluten is a combination of two reactive proteins, gliadin and glutenin, which are present in wheat, barley, and rye. It helps give bread its chewy texture and elasticity.

But it's not just found in breads. Gluten is used as an additive in processed foods, a thickening agent in soups and sauces, a fermenting agent in condiments, beer, and grain alcohols, a binding agent in medications . . . I could go on, but in simple terms: Gluten is everywhere. (See the hidden sources of gluten list at: wholelifenutrition.net/learn/gluten-free.)

CASE STUDY

I will never forget Haley, a beautiful 2-year-old girl who came into my clinical practice in 2006. She was suffering from bouts of terrible bloody stools that would have her parents rushing her off to the children's

---

hospital multiple times a month. I had suspected food sensitivities, and her parents tried a grain-free and dairy-free elimination diet. The bloody stools stopped.

After Haley's intestines had been calm for quite some time, her mother wanted to reintroduce grains back into her diet and asked what I would recommend. I suggested rice, quinoa, or millet. She went to the local co-op, grabbed some millet from the bulk bin, and served it up for dinner. Haley went right back to the children's hospital.

Frustrated with myself, I went to the co-op to see what was wrong. I poured some millet into a plastic bag and sifted through it with my fingers. Sure enough, I saw some grains in there that did not look like they belonged. Upon closer examination, I saw that they were wheat kernels. Further investigation revealed that lentils, oats, millet, sorghum, and buckwheat are often cross-rotated with gluten-containing crops in the fields. This means that the farmers will rotate the planting of gluten-containing crops on the same land as the gluten-free crops. This leads to a frequent cross contamination with gluten on those products as they are commonly harvested, stored, transported, and processed on the same machinery.

As long as Haley avoided all grains except quinoa and rice, her symptoms subsided.

The problem with the ubiquity of gluten is that it has an exceptional ability to cause irritation. That's because it can't be broken down properly by human digestion. Instead of reaching your small intestines in tiny groups of amino acids called di- and tripeptides (made up of 2 or 3 amino acids each), gluten is left in larger peptide fragments that are highly troublesome to immune cells.

World-renowned research scientist and gluten expert from Massachusetts General Hospital Dr. Alessio Fasano says that the prime issue with gluten is the shape it maintains. He states that no one on this planet digests it well, and our immune cells mistake the undigested peptides from gluten as being a dangerous bacteria. Either directly or indirectly, these peptides can trigger a release of potent inflammatory chemicals called cytokines from the immune cells. These inflammatory cytokines act both locally and globally.

Locally, they can damage the intestinal wall (particularly when genetics for celiac disease are present) and disrupt digestive processes.

Globally, the inflammatory chemicals released by the intestinal immune cells can travel into the bloodstream. Increased levels of these inflammatory chemicals circulating in the bloodstream have been associated with type 2 diabetes, obesity, arthritis, migraine, Alzheimer's, heart disease, and eczema, among other conditions.

Gluten has an amazing ability to break down the defenses of your intestinal wall. It can bind to your intestinal cells and causes them to release a protein called zonulin. Zonulin is an important gatekeeper responsible for opening up junctions between your intestinal cells to allow particles to pass through. We don't want zonulin released constantly in the intestines. Gaps here let food particles and trillions of organisms escape into the blood, and contribute to leaky gut syndrome. This could be happening to you after every meal.

A 2006 article in the *Scandinavian Journal of Gastroenterology* indicated that *all* people will get at least a mild case of leaky gut after eating gluten. If someone has a healthy intestinal tract with calm immune cells, friendly organisms, and nonreactive genetics, this leaky gut will close in a short period of time with little harm done. If someone has hyperactive immune cells, harmful organisms, and/or **celiac disease** or even **non-celiac gluten sensitivity**, this leaky gut can be a real problem.

Celiac Disease

Gluten can cause an incurable (but treatable) autoimmune condition called celiac disease, which is estimated to affect approximately 1 in 100 people. Nearly all of those who develop celiac disease have the genetic predisposition to do so. But genes alone don't mean that the disease will develop; usually a trigger or trauma switches the disease on. Surgery, infection, childbirth, the death of a spouse, vitamin deficiency, and bacterial imbalances all have been shown to contribute to someone manifesting celiac disease. A 2013 study published in *Nutrients* confirmed that stress of the system could leave a person more likely to develop celiac disease. Researchers from the University of Salerno, Italy, wrote, "adults with celiac disease reported more frequent and more severe life events in the years prior to the diagnosis than control patients."

WILL ALL PEOPLE WITH
THE CELIAC GENE DEVELOP
THE DISEASE?

No. Up to 30 percent of the general population actually carries the genes for celiac disease, but only 3 percent with these gene variants will develop the disease. It appears that celiac disease, along with most autoimmune diseases, needs 3 factors in order to manifest: the genes, an environmental trigger (e.g., gluten), and a leaky gut. When we look at the fact that there has been a 5-times increase in cases of celiac disease in the last sixty years, we know that this troublesome trifecta is occurring more often.

There are reasons for this unprecedented rise in cases. Increases in chemical pollutants in our environment and heavy use of antibiotics have proven to change our immune cell function, which can contribute to how we react or overreact to foods. Antibiotics also kill beneficial microbes in our bodies that help our immune cells to remain calm, and keep our intestinal tracts healthy so that leaky gut doesn't develop.

Researchers are suggesting that celiac disease will continue to affect more people as developing lives are exposed to greater levels of environmental insults. Writing in *Advances in Medicine* in 2014, Dr. Rodney Dietert from Cornell University addressed the challenges a child will have developing their immune system in the modern world, including the chemical exposure in the womb that can shift immune cells to be more reactive.

The end result is a higher likelihood that our immune cells may react to gluten in our food supply. It doesn't help that we're also consuming more wheat in processed foods, and that modern wheat varieties have been bred to contain more gluten. Wheat today is drastically different from what we were eating forty years ago; it's been hybridized to be shorter in length and have much larger wheat kernels. While this has benefited the agricultural businesses by producing more yields, it has left us with wheat varieties that are difficult to digest and loaded with potentially irritating compounds.

When you have celiac disease, your immune system starts attacking your own intestinal cells. This leads to constant inflammation, a leaky gut, nutrient deficiencies, and an imbalance in the organisms found in the intestinal tract. When these 4 factors are present, several other diseases can begin to develop. In fact, researchers have associated more than 200 diseases with celiac disease.

While researchers estimate that around 1 percent of the population suffers from celiac disease, an article in *Post Graduate Medicine Journal* in 2006 stated a staggering observation: "Population-based screening studies suggest that as many as 50–90% of people with celiac disease...are living undiagnosed in the community."

In my own clinical practice, I commonly see clients who were diagnosed with a multitude of other issues before they were finally diagnosed with celiac disease. On average, it takes them ten years to get an accurate diagnosis. That's not a misprint. Typically, people have seen numerous doctors, taken handfuls of medications, and suffered for countless days before they finally go on a gluten free diet and feel like a million bucks.

Doctors used to think celiac disease was very rare and only looked for diarrhea, nutrient deficiencies, and weight loss to diagnose it. When they saw these symptoms, they would request a biopsy where a sample of the upper intestines was examined under a microscope. If the intestinal biopsy revealed that the hairlike cells of the intestines—the villi, which help absorb nutrients from food—were eroded down to stubs or holes (a condition known as Marsh III villous atrophy), then you were diagnosed with celiac disease.

But this process was flawed because it assumed two things: 1) that the majority of symptoms that occur with celiac disease and other gluten-related disorders occur in the intestines, and 2) that a negative biopsy guarantees a person doesn't have celiac disease. These assumptions left millions of people in a sort of medical no-man's-land with no clear diagnosis or treatment plan.

In reality, symptoms of celiac disease are likely to spring up all over the body. In my own practice and research, the following conditions and symptoms have presented a link to celiac disease:

Skin disorders: eczema, acne (rosacea and vulgaris), psoriasis, atopic dermatitis, dermatitis herpetiformis

Mental disorders: anxiety, depression, atypical bipolar disorder, eating disorders

Respiratory and sinus disorders: asthma, rhinitis, sinusitis, nasal polyps

Gastrointestinal disorders: GERD, diarrhea, constipation, gas, nausea, bloating, intestinal cramping, sharp pains in the abdomen

Sleep disorders: insomnia, sleep apnea

Neurological disorders: autism spectrum disorders, Parkinson's disease, multiple sclerosis, numbness and tingling in the hands and feet, Raynaud's disease, one side of the face going numb after eating gluten, memory loss, ataxia

Metabolic disorders: type 2 diabetes, metabolic syndrome, obesity, failure to thrive, elevated cholesterol, excessively low cholesterol

Aches and pains: chronic back and neck pain, migraines, rheumatoid arthritis, unexplained joint pains

Bone disorders: osteoporosis, osteomalacia, osteopenia

Nutrient deficiencies: vitamin D, iron, zinc, folates, magnesium, calcium, vitamin K, tryptophan, phenylalanine, and vitamin B12

Only when gluten was removed were clients able to see symptoms and conditions such as these improve or subside.

If you are experiencing chronic diarrhea, persistent weight loss, iron deficiency anemia, osteoporosis, or other symptoms that are nonresponsive to treatment, you can ask your doctor to run a test for celiac disease.

Today, there are multiple ways to get tested. Numerous articles have shown that the old gold standard, taking a tissue biopsy from the upper intestinal tract, can produce false negatives. Some have theorized that this is because the person being tested has intestinal symptoms in a place that is not sampled in the biopsy. So they've recommended that up to four or more biopsy samples be taken to avoid this issue, which can be quite invasive and expensive.

Thankfully, there are blood tests available now that look at four different markers and are coming close to replacing a biopsy. Those markers are for four different types of antibodies. Research published in *BMC Gastroenterology* in January 2013 found that when all four are present, there is a 99 to 100 percent chance of predicting celiac disease.

(In case you want to request these tests from your doctors, the antibodies referred to in the study were named IgA anti-deamidated gliadin peptides (dpgli), IgG anti-dpgli, IgA anti-tissue transglutaminase, and IgA anti-endomysium.)

If you test positive for celiac disease, the treatment is to avoid gluten completely. While there is no cure for celiac disease, this treatment is highly effective—once they remove gluten from their diets, most people feel infinitely better in a very short period of time.

Remember that a negative test for celiac does not mean you don't have it or that you don't fall somewhere else along the spectrum of gluten reactivity. Many of my clients who've benefited from removing gluten were without the genetics or a positive biopsy for celiac disease. The best test is to follow the Elimination Diet and see how you feel when you remove gluten from your diet and then add it back.

EATING GLUTEN-FREE

If you've been diagnosed with celiac disease or gluten sensitivity, rejoice! Now that you know what is causing all your crazy symptoms, you can avoid years of suffering unnecessarily. Trust me. This is a great thing. Now, here is the next great thing: Eating gluten-free is delicious! And it can be extremely healthy, too. Just beware of all the processed "gluten-free products" on the market, many of which are filled with ingredients that will not bring you optimal health, and may not truly be gluten-free. To safeguard your health, I highly suggest you call the manufacturers of gluten-free foods and ask them these simple questions:

Do you have a dedicated gluten-free facility?
If not, what steps do you take to avoid cross contamination?
Have you contacted your raw material suppliers and made sure their ingredients are batch tested for gluten content?
Do you batch test all of your products to guarantee they are indeed gluten-free?

Along with a client of mine, I called more than 150 manufacturers of gluten-free foods and asked these very questions. Only **10** answered these questions to my satisfaction. Indeed, I have many clients who are eating foods that are not truly gluten-free and who never really get better. If you examine the research and clinical observations, many products with millet, lentils, oats, sorghum, and buckwheat will not truly be gluten-free.

This tells you that the potential for gluten contamination is great. You will need some help identifying hidden sources and navigating the wonderful world of gluten-free cooking. This book includes plenty of gluten-free recipes for you to enjoy, and you can also turn to our website (WholeLifeNutrition.net), our blog (NourishingMeals.com), and our cookbooks (*Whole Life Nutrition Cookbook* and *Nourishing Meals*).

Non-Celiac Gluten Sensitivity (NCGS)

For a period of time, those who fell into the gray area of gluten reactivity did so without a medically defined condition. I consulted many of these individuals who seemed to belong to a unique population of gluten-sensitive people without a celiac diagnosis. They had what looked and acted like celiac disease from the outside but all of their blood tests and biopsies came back negative. And yet when they took the gluten out of their diet, they got better.

This "not full-blown celiac disease" is called gluten sensitivity. An article in *Digestion and Liver Disorders* in 2003 and another in *Gastroenterology* in 1980 revealed that there indeed was an entity other than celiac disease out there. And only in the last few years have researchers begun to address NCGS as its own entity.

Up to 6 percent of the general population suffers from NCGS, and the symptoms associated with it are almost as extensive as celiac disease. Here are common symptoms experienced by those with gluten sensitivity:

- Bloating
- Crankiness, anxiety, depression
- Diarrhea
- Eczema
- Fatigue
- Foggy thinking
- Gas

- Intestinal irritation
- Joint pains
- Migraines
- Mood problems
- Nausea
- Reflux/GERD

We've discussed the elements of gluten that have been linked to celiac disease. But according to "Non-celiac gluten sensitivity. Is it in the gluten or the grain?" a review published in the *Journal of Gastrointestinal and Liver Diseases*, there are other irritating characteristics present in gluten that can cause NCGS and increase inflammation in healthy individuals:

- **Lectins:** Gluten contains lectins, carbohydrate-binding proteins found in seeds and grains that protect them from fungi and competitive plants. The specific lectin compounds in wheat, wheat germ agglutinin (WGA), have been shown to cause a release of inflammatory chemicals from intestinal immune cells, and may contribute to a leaky gut as well. As mentioned earlier, a high concentration of WGA also could lower the pancreas's ability to produce digestive enzymes by 70 percent.
- **Alpha-amylase/trypsin inhibitors** (ATIs): Found in wheat and other gluten-containing grains, ATIs directly stimulate immune cells to secrete inflammatory chemicals.
- **Fructans:** Wheat is specifically high in fructans, starches that are not easily broken down by humans and may feed the bacteria involved in small intestinal bacterial overgrowth (SIBO).

Because there's currently no laboratory test to accurately diagnose this disorder, you must let your symptoms guide you—if you are experiencing any of the symptoms listed beginning on page 56, you might have non-celiac gluten sensitivity. The only way you can find out if you have this is to eliminate gluten during the Elimination Diet. If your symptoms return when you add gluten back in, then you will have clearly identified the root of the problem.

Could you continue to eat gluten even if your Elimination Diet experiment reveals it as the source of your symptoms? You could, but you should know the risks involved. If your immune system is reacting to gluten every time you eat, and you continue to eat gluten, research has indicated you are more likely to suffer from disease. Liver cancer rates can go up; your risk of dying may increase by 600 percent compared to those who choose not to eat gluten; and your rate of autoimmune disease may increase. In essence, if you are having a constant smoldering of inflammation due to gluten consumption, you are more susceptible to most modern diseases.

Dairy

Clients don't like me when I mention the need to remove dairy during the Elimination Diet. Everyone loves milk, cheese, butter, ice cream, and other dairy-containing foods, so I usually have to present a solid and compelling case for cutting them out. It's not a tough case to build—here are six reasons dairy could be disrupting your digestion and damaging your health.

1. **Lactose:** For starters, cow's milk contains lactose, a type of sugar that is not well tolerated by most adults: Between 60 and 75 percent of adults can't properly digest it. Most of us no longer produce lactase, the enzyme needed to break down lactose. Symptoms of lactose intolerance can be mild to severe and include: cramping, bloating, abdominal pain, diarrhea, and vomiting.
2. **Mucus:** Most milk contains a protein by the name of BCM 7. This protein is known to increase mucus production in the respiratory and digestive systems in animals. A 2010 article in *Medical Hypothesis* by Bartley and McGlashan suggested that this byproduct of milk breakdown may create excess mucus production in people. Excess mucus can worsen upper respiratory issues such as asthma and decrease nutrient absorption in the gut.
3. **Insulin spikes:** Milk has a high insulinogenic effect. When you drink it, your pancreas triggers the release of a ton of insulin. High levels of insulin promote inflammation, which we are directly working to minimize with the Elimination Diet.
4. **Toxin pollutants:** Dairy products have been proven to contain some of the highest concentrations of environmental pollutants such as

flame retardants and dioxins. Research from both *Environmental Health Perspectives* in 2010 and the *Journal of Toxicology and Environmental Health* in 2001 indicate these toxins can damage the immune system, and long-term exposure can lead to reproductive and developmental problems.

Toxins end up in dairy and other foods by way of bioaccumulation and biomagnification, processes that occur in the natural world. When chemicals like dioxins are released into the air, they will settle on the plants and soil. Plants will accumulate more dioxins over time. Animals that eat those plants will accumulate even larger amounts of dioxins. Because persistent organic pollutants (POPs) such as dioxins, PCBs, PBDEs, and DOT bind to fat, they will be stored in fat tissues and freed when an animal uses that stored fat to make milk for their offspring.

The breast-feeding offspring will get up to 25 percent of that animal's fat accumulating toxins through the milk of their mother. In other words, the amount of toxins is magnified when passed through the milk. When we consume cow's milk frequently, we are taking the place of the calf in receiving the accumulated toxins from the cow.

5. **Chemicals and hormones:** When Spanish and Moroccan researchers tested the chemical content of milk in 2010, they were shocked to discover 20 "pharmacologically active substances." Their findings were published in the *Journal of Agriculture and Food Chemistry* and showed evidence of contamination of the milk by antibiotics, antifungal medications, anti-inflammatories, and hormones, such as estrogen. You're probably wondering how this is even possible. Well, some of the medications were given directly to the cows, some were applied to the udders and migrated into the milk, but other traces were linked to diet (cattle food) and environment. Many of these medications can damage your gut and lead to bacterial imbalances.

6. **Disrupted digestion:** Cow's milk contains protease inhibitors, which can create or worsen leaky gut. These inhibitors prevent enzymes from digesting proteins. Undigested proteins can activate the immune system, setting off the inflammation cascade that can cause leaky gut.

CORN AND SOY

Removing gluten and dairy from your diet are a great starting point, but the most accurate and efficient way to identify the source of discomfort within your unique system is to remove all possible sources of irritation. Only when we remove all reactive foods can we create a blissfully calm gut. And this is the ultimate key to your complete recovery. Dr. Sidney Baker, one of the founders of Functional Medicine and the Autism Research Institute, always says, "If you are sitting on two tacks and you take one out, do you feel 50 percent better?" It is necessary to remove all of your irritating foods in order to get to a state of calm.

Corn

Like gluten, corn is everywhere. It's not just when you know you're eating corn that you're consuming it—there are hundreds of corn-derived ingredients hidden in processed foods, the most well-known and prevalent being high-fructose corn syrup.

What do we have against this favorite summertime vegetable? First off, it's not a vegetable at all; it's a grain that has similar protein structures to gluten. And this means just like gluten, it contains inflammatory properties. Corn is full of prolamins, the same plant storage proteins found in other grains that are resistant to digestion in the human body.

Here's the other trouble with corn: Nearly all the corn in the United States comes from genetically modified seeds. And more than 85 percent of the crops are grown from a seed that's been engineered to produce its own insecticide. This type of corn contains a type of Bt-toxin that kills bugs by poking holes in their intestines.

Producers of Bt-toxin seeds have claimed that the pesticide doesn't impact humans. And yet researchers writing in *Reproductive Toxicology* in 2011 presented a different truth. Canadian researchers tested pregnant and non-pregnant women and found evidence of Bt-toxin in:

- 93 percent of maternal blood samples
- 80 percent of fetal blood samples
- 69 percent of non-pregnant women blood samples

Research is still being conducted to reveal the impact of elements such as Bt-toxin on our health. Still, there are other modifications made to genetically modified organism (GMO) crops that make them genuine digestion disturbers. By design, they are made to be more resistant to pests. This resistant nature carries over to your digestive system, where GMO foods will resist being broken down by enzymes. Undigested food particles can produce symptoms of allergy and sensitivity, and increase the chances of developing leaky gut.

By eliminating corn, you will also be removing one of the most insidious and damaging foods: corn sugar, otherwise known as high-fructose corn syrup (HFCS). HFCS has zero nutritional benefits and may contribute to a leaky gut, and the chronic consumption of HFCS can increase your risk for fatty liver disease.

According to Dr. Lyn Patrick, an expert on liver disorders with the American College for the Advancement of Medicine, it only takes the consumption of 25 to 35 grams of fructose in one sitting to lead someone on the path to disease.

Here's how the pathway can develop: When high levels of fructose are consumed at one time, the body cannot absorb and process it fast enough. The extra fructose lingers in the intestines where it will feed bacteria, allowing them to grow rapidly. These bacteria can irritate the intestines, leading to a leaky gut, which will allow bacteria to sneak into the blood and increase inflammation. The inflammatory chemicals can then travel to the liver and cause damage.

Along with our normal use in candy, sauces, and processed foods, the consumption of HFCS in flavored coffee beverages sweetened with syrup and in sodas has led to a massive increase in fructose consumption. How much flavored/syrup-sweetened coffee would you have to drink to ingest 25 to 35 grams of fructose? Just look at the sugar content of your sweetened coffee beverage and divide that by half. Most sweetened syrups are made with high-fructose corn syrups that are 55 percent fructose. A popular 16-ounce, vanilla-flavored coffee beverage with whipped cream has almost 70 grams of sugar and 35 grams of fructose. Drinking one of those a day for three months or longer can leave you more susceptible to fatty liver disease.

Fructose beyond 20 to 25 grams at a time can also lead to intestinal distress. The extra fructose is rapidly fermented by bacteria in the upper intestines, leading to gas, bloating, distension, and what my clients call "gooey poops." If these bacteria are fed often, they can overgrow and irritate the intestinal wall.

FRUCTOSE MALABSORPTION

If you have irritable bowel, loose bowels, cramping, diarrhea, and excessive gas, you may want to lower your intake of fructose while on the Elimination Diet. Certain fruits are relatively high in fructose, including apples, pears, cherries, watermelon, and mangoes. Approximately 30 percent of all people diagnosed with irritable bowel syndrome (IBS) have been shown to have a hard time digesting fructose and are thus said to have fructose malabsorption.

And we already know that repeated damage to the lining of the gut will cause leaky gut, allowing particles and toxins to float freely into the bloodstream and increasing inflammation. Since we are working to heal the gut and reduce inflammation with the Elimination Diet, corn must fall strictly on the "no" list during the program.

Soy

Soybean or soy is a type of legume that is eaten whole as edamame, or processed into other forms you might be familiar with: tofu, tempeh, and soy milk. In lesser-known forms, it is used as an additive in processed foods. You might see it on a label as soybean oil, hydrolyzed soybean protein, soy albumin, or soy lecithin. This last one is in nearly all packaged cookies and candies.

Like corn and gluten, soy is sneaky. It's in baked goods, deli meats, protein bars, cereal, chicken broth, mayonnaise, vitamins, peanut butter, sauces, soups, and more. Eating a diet of whole, fresh foods is pretty much the only way to avoid soy.

Also like corn, much of the soy in the United States (94 percent) is genetically modified. In fact, soy was the first major genetically modified crop in 1996, having been modified to withstand excessive spraying of the herbicide Roundup. A 2014 article in *Food Chemistry* entitled "Compositional differences in soybeans on the market: Glyphosate accumulates in Roundup Ready GM soybeans" showed that not only are these genetically modified soy plants less nutritious than their conventional counterparts, but they are also laden with herbicide residues.

Soy is naturally resistant to digestive enzymes produced by the pancreas. It produces compounds that inhibit the pancreatic enzyme trypsin from breaking down proteins in foods (hence their name, trypsin inhibitors). Genetically modified soy has been found to have higher amounts of these inhibitors, making it even more difficult to digest. If we do not break down the proteins found in foods, we are more likely to have immune reactions to those foods.

ADDITIONAL REACTIVE FOODS

When you get to the phases of the Elimination Diet, you'll notice that you will be removing foods beyond gluten, dairy, soy, and corn. Every food that is removed is done so with specific purpose. Each item that appears on the "no" list has the potential to irritate or inflame your unique system. As we work to create the most calm, peaceful intestinal environment for you, all of these potential contributors must be removed. Failing to do so could create inaccurate results during the Reintroduction Phase or, worse, ensure that your symptoms stay put.

Here are a number of the other foods on the removal list and their most irritating characteristics:

Alcohol

You'll want to avoid alcohol during the Elimination Diet. Beer, wine, and hard alcohol aren't kind to your gut, and drinking them will hinder your efforts to create a calm intestinal environment. This does not mean you have to quit drinking forever, but it does mean you're in for a dry spell if you truly want relief from your symptoms.

What about just one drink? The science advises you against it. Gin, vodka, whiskey, and beer may have gluten proteins in them. One little sip and your entire experiment may be thrown off. Besides, even the slightest bit of alcohol may create micro damage to the villi of the small intestines. It actually burns the sensitive tips of the villi, which are important for secreting digestive enzymes and absorbing important nutrients. If the alcohol contains gluten, even more damage can be done.

When alcohol is drunk in excess or on an empty stomach, it can accelerate the development of leaky gut. It seems to have a unique ability to open gaps for endotoxins, which are bacterial compounds that cause inflammation and damage tissue.

Alcohol will also feed bad bacteria, increasing the risk of bacterial overgrowth or an imbalanced gut environment.

Beef

Beef proteins have been shown to have cross-reactivity with dairy proteins in some individuals. This means that people who are really dairy sensitive may not tolerate beef. In multiple articles on rheumatoid arthritis and the elimination diet, both Kicklin et al. and Darlington et al. found that beef was one of the top irritant foods for arthritis. And when Dr. Ellen Grant of Charing Cross Hospital in London tested foods and their effect on allergies, beef was found to be one of the top contributors to migraines.

Pork

Pork is the second most common food irritant found in gallbladder disease. People who regularly consume bacon, lard, and other pork products may start reacting to the pork proteins found in these products. Reactions can be experienced as stomach pain, bloating, excessive gas, cramping, and constipation.

According to Zar and Benson in the *American Journal of Gastroenterology* in 2005, antibodies to pork were found to be significantly higher in subjects with irritable bowel syndrome as well.

Avoiding beef, pork, and all processed meats during the Elimination Diet will ensure that you aren't exposed to nitrites, to which many people can be sensitive. These commonly used food additives can cause headaches, fatigue, runny nose, and even hives, if you're allergic.

Chocolate and Coffee

Chocolate and coffee both contain chemicals called methyl xanthines (theobromide in chocolate; caffeine in coffee). These molecular compounds can contribute to anxiety, sleeplessness, and heart palpitations in people. When someone is anxious or excited, they can secrete more cortisol, and elevated cortisol can cause a permeable gut.

IgG food sensitivity panels and dietary challenge tests are finding many people react to both coffee and chocolate. Children with anxiety and autism have a particularly high reactivity rate to chocolate.

In 2009, the Autism Research Institute compiled results from more than 25,000 questionnaires filled out by parents of autistic children. The answers determined what interventions, whether they were medical or lifestyle changes, had the most positive effects on their children. The removal of wheat, dairy, and chocolate were among the top four.

Citrus

You've likely heard of the warnings on medications that caution against taking them with grapefruit juice. This is because certain compounds in citrus fruits (naringin and others) have the capacity to alter liver enzymes significantly. If you slow down liver enzyme function, medications, toxins, and other substances are more likely to loiter in the body, ready to irritate and damage cells. As time goes on, I see more and more people starting to react to proteins in citrus as well. Rashes, fatigue, and abdominal pain are three common symptoms of citrus reactions.

Eggs

Eggs are a highly allergenic food, and yet most people would never think to blame them for symptoms such as bloating, gas, nausea, and skin rashes.

Eggs contain an enzyme called lysozyme, which will link up with undigested egg white proteins. Together they'll form what's known as a lysozyme complex. A lysozyme complex will float through the digestive system and resist digestion while picking up bacterial proteins, growing bigger as it travels.

Once at the gut barrier, the complex will slip right through—lysozyme possesses a unique chemical ability to cross through cellular junctions. From here, it maneuvers into the blood where it circulates throughout the body. The undigested proteins will trip the immune cells' alarm, kicking out inflammatory chemicals.

Nightshades

The term *nightshade* actually refers to the Solanaceae family of plants, which includes tomatoes, potatoes, sweet and hot peppers, cayenne and paprika (made from peppers), eggplant, goji berries, and tomatillos. Nightshades found in the wild contain levels of chemicals called alkaloids that prevent us from eating them. The common vegetables we use today have been bred to contain much lower levels of these alkaloids, but some sensitive individuals still react to even small amounts. Those individuals sensitive to nicotine, a common alkaloid in eggplant and tomatoes, may want to eliminate those foods from their diets.

Even if you find that you are not sensitive to nightshades after following the Elimination Diet, be sure to remove the greening and sprouting parts of potatoes. These portions are indicators of an increase in alkaloid compounds, and high concentrations of these can cause problems for most people. Only store your potatoes for up to three weeks in a dark and dry area to prevent them from sprouting and turning green.

Tree Nuts and Peanuts

Tree nuts and peanuts are two of the top eight triggers of food allergies. Examples of tree nuts are cashews, hazelnuts, almonds, pecans, and walnuts. You can be sensitive or allergic to one nut or another, or separately to peanuts, although most people with an allergy to peanuts are also allergic to one or more tree nuts.

There are numerous reasons as to why tree nuts and peanuts are so reactive for many. Here are four of the most likely:

1. They are hard to digest. Nature has designed nuts and seeds to be resistant to digestion by animals so they can be spread across the land in animal fecal matter. They have hard coatings that are difficult to digest, enzyme inhibitors that interfere with digestion, and lectins that may disrupt the intestinal lining.
2. They have a high protein content. Protein fragments from foods (peptides) can be mistaken for foreign invaders by the immune cells if they are not broken down very well during the digestive process. These undigested proteins might mimic a common invader of the

body like rotovirus, for example. Because of this, any food that has high protein content and is not digested well is more likely to stimulate an immune reaction in the intestinal tract, especially if that intestinal tract is "leaky."

3. They often have toxins from mold on them. Peanuts are legumes that grow underground in a moist environment, where there's a risk of mold developing. Most all samples of peanuts in the United States contain traces of a mold toxin known as aflatoxin. This substance, when not properly detoxified, may cause liver damage as well as contribute to cancer risk.

4. They have high anti-nutrient content (phytates and oxalates). Peanuts are particularly good sources of both oxalates and phytates. These are two substances that are known to bind to minerals like zinc and calcium in your foods and make them less available to your body.

Unless nuts are soaked, sprouted, and then dehydrated, digesting nuts can be a challenge for most. Soaking reduces the phytate content of nuts and neutralizes enzyme inhibitors. Still, nuts—soaked or not—are to be avoided during the first two phases of the Elimination Diet, and then added back in strategically during the Reintroduction Phase.

Sesame

In some parts of the world, sesame has landed on the list of top 10 most allergenic foods. This is because sesame has the perfect combination for a potentially reactive food. First off, it's an amino acid–rich protein source, which can make it difficult for people who can't properly digest proteins. It's also a seed, which means by design it will resist being broken down by acids and enzymes due to its hard coating, enzyme inhibitors, and lectins. A seed wants to survive to keep its genes alive. Watch for sesame on breads, buns, and bagels, and in crackers, dips, and spreads.

Sugar

Sugar is sticky. Setting a lollipop on a couch cushion will prove this point quickly. When the concentration of sugar in your blood builds up, the sugar can stick to proteins there. One such protein is called hemoglobin, which you may know as the protein responsible for carrying oxygen through the body. When it has sugar stuck to it, the hemoglobin will be in a different shape.

When hemoglobin proteins change shape, they can't do their job very well. But there is something else that happens when a protein changes shape: It is no longer recognized by immune cells as being normal and not harmful. The immune system will flag the sticky, misshapen proteins as foreign invaders and launch an attack against them. This attack leads to inflammation and all sorts of symptoms.

Beyond that, some people actually have immune-mediated reactions toward sugar—they can have an allergic response. I see this appear on IgG food allergy/sensitivity panels quite often. They might experience symptoms such as rashes, fatigue, and headaches, and never think of sugar as the cause.

It's also important to remove sugar from your diet during the Elimination Diet because most of the sugar in the United States comes from a combination of beets and sugarcane. Both of these crops are known to use high levels of herbicides. The majority of beets used for sugar (95 percent) are genetically modified to withstand herbicides like Roundup and when tested, often have high levels of herbicide residues on them.

Yeast

Some studies have estimated that up to 60 percent of people with a gluten reaction may have a cross-reaction with yeast as well. If you have Crohn's disease, you will have produced antibodies to yeast. Because strains of yeast that live in our intestines may be presented to our immune cells throughout our lives, this is a common substance that people may find they are sensitive to. Yeasts are found in baked goods, alcohols, and nutritional yeast products.

A HEALING DIET, NOT A DEPRIVATION DIET

Don't be overwhelmed by the list of foods in this book—remember, this is about creating a customized diet. You're going to discover which foods work best for you and which don't. I know it can be hard to give up some of your favorite foods, but think about how much better you'll feel once you do! You are going to have to make a decision and ask yourself this question: Do I want the foods or do I want to lose the symptoms? The choice is clear to me, especially when it can be so delicious to follow the diet!

Now that you understood the foods that are the biggest culprits, let's take a look at another key factor: the environment.

4

THE EFFECT OF ENVIRONMENTAL CHEMICALS

People don't often realize the impact environmental chemicals can have on their health. That was the case for Jimmy, a 40-year-old man who came to see me with a mysterious illness. Six months before he contacted me, he had come down with terrible muscle aches and pains, problems breathing, and debilitating fatigue. Almost overnight he had also become sensitive to many foods and had unpredictable bowel movements. Although he was extremely tired all the time, he just couldn't seem to get restful sleep. All his symptoms were sudden and mysterious, and they showed no signs of letting up.

He was proactive in seeking help. He had gotten expensive laboratory work-ups and evaluations that he shared with a handful of physicians, and not one could pinpoint the origin of his problems. Some even suggested that it was all in his head.

Within 20 minutes of our first conversation, I stopped him and asked: "So...when did you remodel your house?" Even though he did not mention remodeling his house, I knew, without a doubt, that he had. Shocked, he said, "A little over six months ago." Precisely when his symptoms had started.

It turned out Jimmy's house was an older one, and he had redone the paint, flooring, and numerous other tasks. I asked, "Is there any time in the last six months that you have felt better?" He said that there had been a weeklong period when he had gone camping, and he noticed his symptoms started to clear up then. This confirmed it for me: It was his house. The chemical exposure to the paints, adhesives, flooring, and everything else he had used to remodel were too much for his system to process.

I suggested that he eliminate some of the irritating foods in his diet and add in lots of fresh, antioxidant-rich vegetables and fruits, as well as some specific supplements for detoxification and mitochondrial function. At the same time, I recommended some ways he could minimize the effects of the chemicals he may have been exposed to in his house. He got an air purifier that would remove volatile organic compounds and opened his windows frequently. Within a few weeks, he started to turn the corner. Within a few months, he was 70 percent better. The food sensitivities disappeared.

How did I know what was wrong with Jimmy? It was a combination of years of dedicated research on the topic of chemical exposure and a fortuitous discovery of the work of Dr. Claudia Miller, an allergist, immunologist, and tenured professor at the University of Texas School of Medicine at San Antonio. Dr. Miller had reported on many case studies where the symptoms had been identical to that of Jimmy's. In her patients, the cause was always an acute exposure to chemicals. The key giveaways were the trouble breathing and the almost overnight development of sensitivities to foods.

Dr. Miller has been examining the effects of exposure on immune function and the rise in sensitivity related disease for the last few decades. In 1996, she coined the term "toxicant-induced loss of tolerance," or TILT, after observing that subjects exposed to chemicals started reacting to many things in their environment. After chemical accidents in the workplace, for example, people would literally develop food sensitivities overnight.

What happens with TILT is the behavior of the immune cells is changed by chemical exposure. The primary job of the immune system is to survey our internal environment and tolerate the vast majority of things with which it comes in contact. We do not want to be reacting to foods, pet dander, pollen, or our very own cells. When our chemical exposure is increased, our immune cells lose their tolerance and start attacking normally harmless substances.

In most of Dr. Miller's case studies, and in the case of Jimmy, the cause was pinpointed to an acute type of chemical exposure. But it's likely that consistent, everyday exposure to pesticides, air pollutants, skincare chemicals, plastics, food additives, and other industrial compounds could have a cumulative effect on the average person. It's also likely that this exposure is at least partly to blame for the rise in food reactions and symptoms of discomfort. What's our chemical exposure like today? Off the charts.

WE'RE ALL OVEREXPOSED

During the last thirty years, the use of environmental chemicals has increased dramatically. The average person living today will inhale air pollutants, ingest pesticide residue, apply chemicals from lotions to his or her skin, eat chemical additives in processed foods, and more. The worst part is, these chemicals are all invisible, and yet they are literally everywhere.

We currently have more than 83,000 chemicals being used in the United States, with well over 74 billion pounds (yes, *billion*) being imported or produced in the United States every single day. That's more than 250 pounds per person per day! (The numbers have grown so high that in May 2011, the American Academy of Pediatrics issued a warning letting average citizens know that government regulations aren't doing much regulating, and that many of these chemicals put our pregnant mothers and infants at risk.)

Recent data show that these chemicals are, without a doubt, contributing to our pandemic rise in disease. In 2011, a team of researchers in Switzerland published an article in the *Annual Reviews of Physiology* that linked chemicals to altered metabolism of sugar and fats. These types of alterations, they shared, could be making us more prone to diabetes and obesity. Other research conducted by Dr. Stephen Genuis of the University of Alberta and published in the *Journal of Environment and Public Health* demonstrated how chemicals are changing our immune system functions and increasing our risk for allergies, asthma, and eczema.

Two scientists with the Harvard School of Public Health, Dr. Grandjean and Dr. Landrigan, also studied the negative effects of chemicals, focusing on their impact on children. They have now classified 11 common chemicals in our environment as neurotoxins capable of damaging the developing minds of our future generations. These included: lead, methylmercury, polychlorinated biphenyls (PCBs), arsenic, toluene, manganese, fluoride, chlorpyrifos, dichlorodiphenyltrichloroethane (DDT), tetrachloroethylene, and polybrominated diphenyl ethers (PBDEs).

The bottom line is that there's a long list of diseases and conditions being linked to chemical exposure, and I suspect this list will only grow longer.

CHEMICALS AND FOOD INTOLERANCE

Because our goal with the Elimination Diet is to create a peaceful, calm internal environment, we have to consider the impact of environmental chemicals and their potential to set you up for food reactions. The focus is often placed on inflammation and its connection to food intolerance, which I talked about in chapter 1. But the reality is that inflammation is merely a response or reaction of the immune cells to harmful invaders. When the immune cells are hyperreactive to *harmless* substances such as food particles, something is programming them to behave that way; the chemicals are causing TILT.

Chemicals will change the behavior of the immune system directly and indirectly. Directly, toxins such as mercury can damage immune cells, causing a change in their function. Toxins can also damage other cells of the body, requiring the immune cells to step in and help clean up the mess with inflammatory chemicals (a sort of "fight fire with fire" situation). Either way, the result is a change in the immune system response and an overall increase in inflammation. Indirectly, toxins can do two primary things: They can kill beneficial microbes and they can interfere with nutrients in our bodies.

Many toxic chemicals like heavy metals, pesticides, chloramine (in drinking water), hand sanitizers, and preservatives kill beneficial bacteria and other microbes that live in our intestinal tracts. As you read in previous chapters, these very same microbes literally train our immune cells how to respond to their environment, so much so that the immune system is being referred to by some scientists as the "microbial interaction system." If we throw the balance of our microbes off by exposing them to chemicals, we will likely throw off the balance of our immune system response.

How does this work? Let's look at the recent data coming out on the herbicide Roundup as an example. Roundup, which is commonly used on GMO crops, is patented as a biocide, meaning it's a known killer of microbes like bacteria. As the most commonly used herbicide on the planet, there are hundreds of millions of pounds of Roundup and chemically similar herbicides applied every year. While scientific articles are just starting to come out about what this might mean for bacteria that come in contact with it, preliminary data does not look good. It appears that glyphosate, the active ingredient in Roundup, can throw off the balance between beneficial and pathogenic microbes.

A 2012 study in *Current Microbiology* showed that bacteria behaved very differently when exposed to Roundup. Bacteria that can cause disease, such as certain salmonella varieties, were shown to be highly resistant to glyphosate, while beneficial bacteria like particular bifidobacterium and lactobacillus species were found to be moderately to highly susceptible to the damaging effects of this herbicide. In other words, many of the good bacteria died when exposed to glyphosate, while some of the bad ones were able to survive. This intestinal imbalance is a recipe for immune system imbalance.

Pesticides and certain chemicals found in medications can also indirectly create overreactive immune cells by lowering vitamin D levels. Vitamin D is one of the most potent immune-calming substances in the human diet. When vitamin D levels are low, you're at greater risk for developing food intolerance and other health issues. A review published in *Mayo Clinic Proceedings* in 2013 associated adequate vitamin D levels with decreasing cancer, diabetes, heart disease, autoimmune diseases, irritable bowel, and muscle pain. Numerous studies have shown how chemicals in medications and pesticides can lower vitamin D levels and cause deficiencies. (Are you getting enough vitamin D? Read more in chapter 5, in the Get Some Sun section beginning on page 99).

The greater your chemical exposure, the more likely you are to stay in the inflamed state and develop food reactions. The upside is you can take steps to curb your exposure starting today, with awareness being the first step. The research and information presented here isn't intended to overwhelm you, but instead to give you the tools to identify where and when you can make changes. In the remainder of this chapter, you'll discover important environmental chemicals to which you should pay attention and some strategies for minimizing exposure. Also be sure to check out chapter 5, where I share recommendations on how to boost your detoxification systems.

ENDOCRINE DISRUPTING CHEMICALS (EDCS)

Many of the chemicals that we are hearing about in the news will disrupt normal hormone functions. Since hormones are made by the endocrine system, these chemicals are named endocrine disrupting chemicals or EDCs. EDCs act as estrogens in the body, contributing to weight gain, immune disorders, and cancers. When a child is exposed to these chemicals in the womb, they will be more likely to have immune cells that will overreact to proteins in the environment, including foods.

Some of the most widely used EDCs are bisphenol-A (BPA) and phthalates; let's explore those a bit further.

Bisphenol-A (BPA): More than 12 billion pounds of BPA are used in industry every year. Originally, BPA was used as a synthetic estrogen that was added to animal feed to fatten them up, which is likely why research has connected tiny exposures to modified fat metabolism in humans. BPA is currently added to plastics to make them pliable and soft. You will find it in the lining of cans, in plastic Tupperware and beverage bottles, and in the coating on grocery store receipts.

Phthalates (pronounced "thal-ates"): These chemical compounds are also added to plastics and can be found in many of the same places as BPA. When used in vinyl flooring, they can leach out into the air and attach to dust particles, which in turn can be inhaled. A 2012 article published in *ASN Neuro* noted that pregnant women exposed to this type of flooring were susceptible to disturbed thyroid function, and their children were more likely to have autism.

Phthalates are also used to fix colors and scents in personal care items (lotions, perfumes, colognes, creams, aftershave, hair gels, and sunscreens) and household items (air fresheners, dryer sheets, and scented candles). They can be absorbed through skin and inhaled. When Dr. Susan Duty and her team at Harvard Public School of Health tested the impact of personal care product use on phthalate levels in 406 men, they found that the use of one single item like cologne or aftershave was shown to increase phthalate levels in the urine by 33 percent.

Reduce Your Exposure:

- **Go natural.** Look for natural ingredient–based organic products that are color-, fragrant-, and phthalate-free. Also make sure the word "parfum" is not on the label.
- **Break a sweat.** When Dr. Genuis and colleagues compared the amount of phthalates eliminated from the body based on the type of elimination—sweat or urine—they found that sweat was superior. In fact, the concentration of phthalates present in sweat was twice as high as that found in urine. Break a sweat today to help clear these toxins from your body. Broccoli sprouts and Epsom salts can also help cleanse the cells and tissues of chemicals (see Life Is Tough: Try Taking a Bath! in chapter 5 on page 99 for more on these strategies).
- **Eat fresh.** A study published in *Environmental Health Perspectives* in 2011 found that eating a "fresh" diet free of canned foods, plastic water bottles, and foods prepared or wrapped in plastic reduced BPA exposure by 66 percent.

PCBS (POLYCHLORINATED BIPHENYLS)

PCBs were used heavily in electrical and industrial materials up until 1979. They were also used in most types of insulation, paints, plastics, and rubber products. Even though many PCBs were banned decades ago, they are still showing up in the blood of many pregnant mothers and the umbilical cord blood of unborn children.

Some PCBs have been found to drastically increase the risk for diabetes (more than 30 times, according to a research published in *Diabetes Care* in 2006), contribute to obesity, increase cancer risk, and reduce fertility. Additionally, researchers with the Department of Neurology at the University of Kentucky determined that PCBs can "disrupt intestinal integrity" and alter gut permeability: prime precursors to leaky gut syndrome.

The most common dietary exposures to PCBs come from fatty fish and unpurified fish oils. You'll also find PCBs in high-fat meats and animal products, but research shows that the greatest source of exposure in people is farmed salmon. In 2014, there was more farmed salmon consumed than beef. Farmed salmon can have more than 40 times the PCBs found in other foods.

Reduce Your Exposure:

- **Go wild.** Consume fish, particularly salmon, labeled "wild caught." Aside from salmon, many other fish stocks are farmed.
- **Trim the fat.** If you can't guarantee that a fish is sourced from the wild, trim all fatty pieces and remove the skin; PCBs accumulate in fatty tissue.
- **Replace old appliances and light fixtures.** TVs, refrigerators, and fluorescent light fixtures made before 1979 can release PCB particles into your home and workplace.

MERCURY FROM FILLINGS AND AIR POLLUTION

In January 2013, delegates from more than 140 different countries met at a convention in Geneva to discuss the dire risks of having too much mercury exposure on planet earth. Hair samples from humans and flesh samples from fish from around the globe are demonstrating that we have passed a safe threshold for mercury in our environment. This mercury can kill beneficial microbes in our intestines (and in our environment), change our immune cell function, alter our digestion, and damage our brains.

Exposures to mercury commonly come from silver amalgam fillings, and predatory fish (see more on fish in chapter 8, in Pick Better Proteins on page 142). The largest source of mercury on the planet comes from air pollution. The burning of coal has caused millions of pounds of mercury to be distributed across the globe in air pollution (14.3 million pounds in 2010 alone).

THE CHEMICAL CLOUD

Did you know that NASA has been tracking something called the Brown Cloud? This is a massive cloud of air pollution that hovers over India and China. It can get pushed up into the jet stream, and within seven days' time, settle over the West Coast of the United States. In fact, Alaskan fisheries are attributing a recent 20 percent rise in fish mercury levels to the increase of pollution in China and India.

There is now twice as much mercury in the top 100 meters of the ocean than there was a century ago, and predatory fish have 12 times the level of mercury in them now compared to preindustrial times.

Reduce Your Exposure:

- **Choose sustainable.** Choose sustainable energy sources by opting for solar or wind power subsidies on your power bills.
- **Check your zinc and selenium intake.** Make sure you are getting optimal zinc and selenium. Zinc is a cofactor for the metallothionine enzyme that can transport mercury out of the body. Selenium is a cofactor for detoxification enzymes (glutathione peroxidase) and other proteins (selenoproteins) that may reduce your risk of damage from mercury.
- **Use sulfur to aid detoxification.** Broccoli sprouts and sulfur-based detox nutrients will assist in increasing the metabolism and excretion of mercury from your body. Read more on these detoxifying strategies in chapter 5.

HAND SANITIZERS (TRICLOSAN) AND SKINCARE PRESERVATIVES (PARABENS)

Many creams, lotions, and sunscreens contain "preservatives," i.e., chemicals that are designed to kill bacteria and other organisms. Two of the most commonly used preservatives in skincare products are parabens and triclosan. Parabens are used to ensure that organisms do not survive in the tube of cream or bottle of lotion. And triclosan is a potent antimicrobial (microbe killer) used in hand sanitizers, lotions, shampoos, and even toothpastes.

Both triclosan and parabens can be absorbed through your skin where they can alter your hormone functions and your immune response to foods. The problem with these substances is they kill many of the beneficial bacteria that are essential to nutrient absorption and digestion.

In 2012, researchers with the Johns Hopkins Division of Allergy and Clinical Immunology set out to determine if there was a link between triclosan and paraben exposure and food sensitivities. After evaluating chemical levels and allergenic responses in more than 800 children, they found that children with elevated levels of triclosan and parabens in their urine had an increase of between 150 and 250 percent in food sensitivities. The change was even more significant in male subjects, who had an almost 400 percent increase. Even when triclosan is discarded into your drinking water, it will kill microbes in the environment, likely some of the same ones that your immune system loves to have around.

Reduce Your Exposure:

- **Opt for thyme instead.** Choose hand sanitizers with thyme oil instead of triclosan. It is more effective and is nontoxic.
- **Check the label.** Look for skin products that say "paraben-free"—if it's not paraben-free, put it back. More brands are moving away from using parabens, so you should be able to find plenty of great options without these toxic preservatives.

FOOD ADDITIVES

Chemical companies have been profiting from the inclusion of artificial sweeteners, food coloring, fillers, and preservatives for almost half a century. As more research comes out, we are seeing how damaging some of these substances can be to our health. (If you want to read more on food additives, I recommend *Rich Food, Poor Food* by Jayson and Mira Calton.)

Tartrazine: Otherwise known as "Yellow Dye Number 5," tartrazine is used in ice cream, candies (no, the yellow color of those gummy bears is not natural), cake mixes, and other processed goods. Tartrazine is one of many food dyes that have been studied for decades, particularly in relation to children's behavior. Studies have suggested connections between food dye consumption and ADHD-like behavior, especially in those who are genetically predisposed to hyperactivity. Additional research by Professor Neil Ward and his team at the University of Surrey in the U.K. connected tartrazine consumption to depletion of zinc, low levels of which have been linked to hyperactive behavior and impaired immune function.

Caramel coloring: This coloring is used primarily in sodas, but you'll also find it in chips, packaged desserts, pickles, and vinegar. Government-sponsored research has shown that caramel coloring consumption is linked to liver, lung, and thyroid cancer in animals. The California Office of Environmental Health Hazard Assessment has listed 29 micrograms as the threshold, given that this is the amount associated with increased cancer risk. And yet certain brands of sodas have been shown to have between 30 and 195 micrograms per can. Some states have moved to eliminate caramel coloring from food and beverages, but keep an eye on what you buy—if you see "caramel coloring" listed as an ingredient, put it back.

Benzoates: Also listed as sodium benzoate and potassium benzoate, these are used as preservatives to prevent processed foods from developing mold and bacteria. When combined with vitamin C, benzoates form benzene, a known cancer-causing chemical.

Brominated vegetable oil (BVO): BVO has been used in a lot of citrus-flavored sodas, sports drinks, and cocktail syrups to prevent separation of the various beverage ingredients. Consuming it in large amounts has led to skin lesions, memory loss, headaches, and fatigue.

Butylated hydroxyanisole (BHA) and butylated hydroxytoluene (BHT): These preservatives often line the walls of packaging used for foods like potato chips, deli meats, cereals, and butter. Food manufacturers are not required to list them on the label when they're used. The National Institutes of Health state that BHA is "reasonably anticipated to be a human carcinogen." And both BHA and BHT are banned in Australia and the U.K. due to their cancer-causing effects.

Reduce Your Exposure:

- **Eat foods without labels.** When you eat only whole, fresh foods, you won't have to worry about any food additives whatsoever! This is really the simplest and most powerful solution to this entire problem.
- **Shop smarter.** Buy foods and products from stores that support healthy ingredients, and always choose organic.
- **Pay attention to labels.** Be a label investigator and keep your eyes peeled for unwanted ingredients, such as the additives shared in this chapter and other chemical names that may be unrecognizable to you.

PESTICIDES

The word *pesticide* literally means "pest-killer." Their primary mode of action is to kill, and we are spraying hundreds of millions of pounds of these killing chemicals on our planet every single year.

Is it possible we are contributing to imbalances in our air, water, soil, food, and bodies by killing organisms with these chemicals? It seems only logical. And yet many chemical companies assure the public that the levels of chemicals are too small to have an effect. I would challenge them to return to the law of physics that states "for every action, there is an equal and opposite reaction," and to read the thousands of articles that point to the fact that many chemicals, especially those that mimic hormones, can work at extremely small doses. In fact, with those that mimic or disrupt hormone function, smaller amounts may be more toxic than larger amounts.

WHEN CHEMICALS ACCUMULATE

Doctors Laura Vandenberg, Theo Colborn, and Tyrone Hayes, along with a robust team of researchers, published two tour-de-force papers—one in *Endocrine Reviews* in June 2012 and one in *Reproductive Toxicology* in July 2013—in which they exposed the errors in our current thinking regarding the safety of endocrine disrupting chemicals. They explained that the current testing for toxicity, which has researchers adding concentrations of chemicals to animals until they demonstrate negative effects, does not work when applied to chemicals that mimic human hormones. In current practices, the tests are conducted with increased doses of the chemicals for only ninety days. The testing reveals nothing about smaller doses over longer periods of time, which is more like how it happens in real life. Most of us are obviously exposed to chemicals for periods much greater than ninety days; we're looking instead at decades of accumulated exposure.

Tiny amounts of these chemicals that mimic hormones circulating in the body will orchestrate thousands of reactions that regulate our mood, energy, and cell growth. They circulate in parts per million, parts per billion, and even parts per trillion. If we have an increase of these hormonal alterations over a long period of time, they could alter our health slowly, taking decades to manifest as cancer, organ damage, or obesity. These researchers ask the obvious question: Why are we only studying short-term toxic effects of chemicals that mimic our hormones?

The most commonly used herbicide on the planet is Roundup, or other herbicides that contain glyphosate, the "active" ingredient in Roundup. In 2008, there were 620,000 tons (1,240,000,000 pounds) of glyphosate produced globally.

For years, Monsanto and other chemical companies have been saying that Roundup and glyphosate are nontoxic and safe enough to drink (residue of these herbicides is regularly found in our water supplies). After a lawsuit filed by the Attorney General of New York against Monsanto in 1996 and numerous scientific studies, the opposite appears to be true. The following have been linked to glyphosate exposure:

- Toxicity in the brain—*Journal of Toxicology* (2014)
- Disruption of male reproductive systems—*Free Radical and Biological Medicine* (2013)
- Disrupted balance of the microbiome—*Current Microbiology* (2013)
- Kidney and liver damage—*Environmental Sciences Europe* (2011)
- Cell malformations—*Chemical Research in Toxicology* (2010)
- Liver damage—*Environmental Toxicology and Pharmacology* (2009)

And the list goes on. What is even more disturbing is how this herbicide works. Roundup works in two ways:

As a **biocidal**, Roundup works to kill off microorganisms in our environment. Animals exposed to glyphosate residue reveal drastic changes in their intestinal microbiome. This is likely because glyphosate doesn't kill pathogenic microbes such as salmonella and clostridium, but does wipe out many of the beneficial species like lactobacillus and bifidobacterium. This leaves a dangerous intestinal imbalance that is vulnerable to disease—and may not just affect animals, but people who eat fruits and vegetables covered in pesticide residue or drink water containing pesticide runoff. Research by Dr. Monika Krüger and her team, published in 2014 in the *Journal of Environmental and Analytical Toxicology*, found that most all animals and people tested had glyphosate in their urine, but this wasn't the surprising part. The study also revealed that "chronically ill humans showed significantly higher glyphosate residues in urine than healthy population." Dr. Nancy Swanson, a published author and ex-physicist for the U.S. Navy, found that as the use of glyphosate went up, so, too, did the rates of many diseases and conditions, including diabetes, obesity, end-stage renal disease deaths, thyroid cancer, and intestinal infections.

The soil is also affected by the sterilizing effects of glyphosate. Dr. Robert Kremer, professor of soil microbiology with the University of Missouri, and others released a paper in 2011 addressing how the increased use of herbicides is responsible for a drastic shift in our soil microorganism content. When life-promoting organisms are absent from soil, plants don't absorb as many nutrients into their roots and are more prone to disease.

As a potent **mineral chelator**, glyphosate binds tightly to essential minerals like manganese, zinc, and calcium, making them unavailable for normal life processes.

It would be bad enough if glyphosate was all we had to consider, but it's not the only chemical found in herbicides such as Roundup. There are others, called surfactants, which damage plant cell walls enough to allow glyphosate to get into the plants. These substances are hundreds, if not thousands, of times more toxic than the glyphosate itself.

Reduce Your Exposure:

- **Eat organic foods and buy only GMO-free foods.** These are essential steps to take; keep reading to discover why.

GENETICALLY MODIFIED FOODS

What is a genetically modified organism or GMO? It is an organism that has a sequence of its DNA changed so it will produce different proteins. After reading hundreds of scientific articles on genetically modified foods and pesticides (like Roundup) associated with genetically modified (GM) foods, I am confused as to how these ever got approved to enter into our food supply. And many interviews with renowned geneticists and plant pathologists later, I am convinced it was, in fact, a very bad decision.

For more information, science, interviews, and videos on GMOs, visit our website at WholeLifeNutrition.net/learn/gmo-free. You will find that there are documented lawsuits demonstrating that even our own FDA scientists did not think these foods were safe and see papers that are now showing that GM crops are not "substantially equivalent" to their non-GM counterparts, which is what the public had been lead to believe.

You will also find data revealing that the pests that were once repelled by GM plants are now resistant to their effects; and that many weeds are resistant to the pesticides being sprayed on GM crops. Even the brightest and best engineers can't outsmart nature for long. In the meantime, we've saturated much of the globe with millions of pounds of herbicides that increase kidney disease, birth defects, brain damage, and a long list of other conditions with unconfirmed, but suspected links.

What's worse is that GM foods are all over our food supply. It is estimated that between 70 and 80 percent of all our processed foods contain genetically modified ingredients, with many of these confirmed to have scientifically unsafe levels of pesticides on them. Soy, corn, cottonseed, and canola have been documented as having high concentrations.

Roundup is the most commonly used herbicide on GM crops. The statistics show that the colossal increase in the use of Roundup is tied directly to the rise of genetically modified crops. From 1996 (when GM crops were introduced) until 2010, there was a:

- 1,427 percent increase in glyphosate application to corn and soy crops
- 1,000 percent increase in intestinal infection death rate
- 550 percent increase in chronic constipation incidence rate
- 205 percent increase in irritable bowel syndrome incidence rate

Similarly, the vast majority of the agricultural crops produced in the United States are now genetically modified to withstand direct spraying with large amounts of Roundup. As a result, they are said to be "Roundup-Ready" (you can see these two are dangerously intertwined):

- Canola (approx. 90 percent of U.S. crop)
- Corn (approx. 88 percent of U.S. crop in 2011)
- Cotton (approx. 90 percent of U.S. crop in 2011)
- Soy (approx. 94 percent of U.S. crop in 2011)
- Sugar Beets (approx. 95 percent of U.S. crop in 2010)

The numbers can make your head spin, and certainly make you wonder if there's any way to avoid GM crops and pesticides. There are ways. The simplest and most straightforward way to minimize your exposure is to buy organic always, or as often as you can.

Reduce Your Exposure:
- **Buy organic** (keep reading for more on organic foods).
- **Buy only 100 percent cane sugar,** if you buy sugar at all.
- **Avoid all soy, corn, cottonseed, and canola oils.**

GOOD-BYE CONVENTIONAL, HELLO ORGANIC

My goal for you is to take the habits you develop during the Elimination Diet and carry them over into your lifestyle long-term—and nothing could be more important than getting into the habit of buying organic foods.

For the sake of letting go of your symptoms, it is essential that you make the commitment to bringing only organic foods into your home. I have witnessed too many clients react to chemically laden, conventionally grown or raised foods not to make this recommendation. In my practice, I have seen the switch to organic foods help children improve their mood and brain function; adults improve arthritis; and countless people experience relief from skin and pain disorders. Many people avoid organic products because of the cost, but that's shortsighted—the costs of eating foods coated in pesticide residue or produced from GM crops will be far greater down the road.

Plenty of the people who come to see me have questions about organic foods, and you might, too. These are the three most common questions I get:

1. Are they really more nutritious?
2. Are they worth the extra cost?
3. Do they really taste better?

The short answer to all three is a resounding "YES!" But let's look a little further into why this is the case.

1. Organic = More Nutrition

It used to be that nutrition was all about protein, carbs, fats, vitamins, and minerals. But we know now that there's a great deal more to consider, namely the biochemical makeup of foods. When we talk about what nourishes the human body best, we have to consider the biochemistry—the messages packed into the foods you eat.

In this department, plants have proven to have the greatest potential to affect our health. Decades of research have revealed that plants are true biochemical wonders, possessing more than tens of thousands of plant chemicals. These chemicals can create profound beneficial shifts in your cells and even alter how your genes are expressed. The field of nutrition is finally paying attention and promoting plants for the stars they are.

But not all plants and the fruits and vegetables they produce are created equal. The environment in which they are grown directly determines how healthy they are for you, or how many of those important beneficial compounds are present. Things like insect bites, weed competition, nutrient changes in the soil, temperature changes, and radiation from sunlight will force a plant to produce protective compounds in order to survive.

Conventional agriculture that uses herbicides, pesticides, and fertilizers is designed to reduce the stress on crops. But these strip away or change all of the natural challenges that will trigger the plant to produce protective compounds. The result: Conventionally grown foods will have less nutrition.

Researchers with Newcastle University in the U.K. confirmed this to be true. After performing an extensive review of the scientific data on conventional and organic produce, Dr. Kirsten Brandt and others found that organic produce indeed had 16 percent higher levels of all protective compounds tested except beta-carotene (this makes sense, as beta-carotene is a natural "sunscreen" for plants and sun exposure does not change in organic versus conventional). The review also cited higher essential amino acids in proteins and higher vitamin C levels in the organic food.

As to be expected, organics were found to consistently contain lower pesticide residues, mycotoxins (toxins produced by fungus growing on the crops), and fewer nitrates (potentially toxic compounds from fertilizer use).

A recent review from Stanford University researchers also concluded that conventionally grown crops show significantly higher residues of pesticides. Additionally, they determined that the practices on conventional farms have contributed to the rise in antibiotic-resistant bacteria.

According to renowned organics expert Dr. Charles Benbrook of Washington State University, the most significant and proven benefits of organic food and farming are:

- A reduction in chemicals that are proven dangerous to developing children
- A healthier balance of omega-6 and omega-3 fatty acids in organic dairy products and meat
- The virtual elimination of industrial practices that create dangerous antibiotic resistant bacteria

When you consider these conclusions alone, my hope is that you will feel motivated to buy and eat only organically grown goods. Still on the fence? There's more.

FOOD FOR THOUGHT

"Over time, I believe that unbiased analysis coupled with modern-day science is likely to show with increasing clarity that growing and consuming organic foods, especially in conjunction with healthy diets rich in fresh, whole foods, is one of the best health-promoting investments we can make today as individuals, families, and a society."

—Dr. Charles Benbrook, research professor at the Center for Sustaining Agriculture and Natural Resources, Washington State University

2. The Price of Chemical-Laden Foods

When you purchase organic foods, you are not only maximizing the amount of nutrition you get from food, you're also voting to reduce the amount of chemicals present in our environment. You are investing in greater health for future generations and helping curb farming practices that threaten each and every one of us.

When conventional farms use pesticides and fertilizers, the residues can build up in waterways and contribute to toxic algal blooms called "red tides." These produce toxins that may kill sea life or poison seafood, making it unsafe for human consumption.

Scientific investigations have also shown that pesticides and fertilizers can have a more direct effect on farmworkers and people who live near application areas. One study found that children whose mothers lived within 500 meters of areas that used pesticides were 4.1 times more likely to develop autism. Those findings were supported by a 2014 paper in *Environmental Health Perspectives* that showed children born to mothers who were within 1,500 meters (just under a mile) from a pesticide spray site were 60 percent more likely to get autism.

A stunning article in the February 2006 edition of *Environmental Health Perspectives* determined that *all* children eating conventional diets in their study had elevated levels of two potent pesticides (malathion and chlorpyrifos) floating around in their blood. When they put these children on organic diets, the levels were almost undetectable within a few days. An April 2011 article in *Time* magazine entitled "Exposure to Pesticides in Pregnancy Can Lower Children's IQ" spoke of how the elevated pesticide levels of these common pesticides has been associated with reflex abnormalities in infants, lower development in 2-year-olds, ADHD-like behaviors in 5-year-olds, and lower IQ scores in 7-year-olds.

Can we afford to pay for organic foods? If we don't make our best effort to do so, the long-term costs in declining health and wellness will be astronomical.

3. Organic Foods Just Taste Better!

Organic foods taste better than conventionally grown foods. You might think it sounds crazy, but it's true. If you have not tried fresh, organic produce, you are in for a real treat! The flavors pop, delivering a clean and pure taste. The texture is completely different—you've never bitten into crunchier carrots or tasted broccoli with a better bite. Your dining experience will improve. The flavors get even better if you can choose locally grown produce from a farmers' market or grow it yourself. Fresh herbs, lettuces, or green beans from a patio planter box will spoil your taste buds for life.

Better nutrition, better taste, better health, and a better planet. Plain and simple . . . organics truly are better.

HOW THE ELIMINATION DIET WILL HELP REDUCE YOUR EXPOSURE

We know that exponential increases in unexplained weight gain, chronic fatigue, depression, irritated bowels, joint pain, and skin problems parallel the increases in our daily chemical exposure. If you are experiencing any of these symptoms, it's especially worth paying attention to your environment and your chemical intake. Don't feel overwhelmed by the need to pay attention, but instead feel empowered by your new awareness.

I hope you'll use many of the steps I've outlined in this chapter to minimize your own chemical exposure. And know, too, that by following the Elimination Diet, you will automatically be drastically reducing your pesticide and food additive intake. Be sure to check out chapter 5 for more on how to maximize detoxification.

PART II

Preparing for the Elimination Diet

5

10 STEPS AND 10 SUPPLEMENTS TO SUPPORT YOU

Now that you know all of the incredible benefits to be had from the Elimination Diet, I hope you're excited to experience them for yourself! My goal is to set you up for success so that you can experience a life free of the symptoms that have plagued you for too long, and feel better than you ever have.

Part of the key to getting the best results out of this program is to be fully prepared before you begin. So before you embark on phase one of the program, this chapter outlines the different types of support that are available to you so you can succeed on the Elimination Diet. Use these support strategies now to help you prepare before you begin the program, and return to them throughout the program to reduce stress and increase calm. Taking these steps in advance of starting the diet will produce great benefits on their own.

As with any new challenge, it's best to build yourself up in order to be better able to take it on—so start applying these supportive and positive steps today to get your momentum and motivation going in the right direction.

1. CREATE A FOOD TRIBE

For the next few months, you will be changing everything you do around food. You will be shopping for new foods, preparing new foods, and eating new foods. All of your normal habits will be replaced by new habits and routines. This can be a really exciting and invigorating time, but it can be a bit overwhelming too. It is best to call in reinforcements!

We have seen the most amazing transformations happen in communities, groups, and families during the Elimination Diet. It appears that there really is power in numbers. The effects of a change in diet and health seem to magnify when there are others with whom to share the experience; people get excited and inspired seeing their friends and colleagues losing weight, experiencing fewer symptoms, and feeling great.

This is why I recommend having a friend, spouse, family member, workout partner, or coworker join you on the Elimination Diet—it really can create a situation that is fun and life affirming. Shopping and cooking can be shared and so can the meals. You can have a person with you who will commiserate about not being able to eat cheese and chocolate, or more important, to celebrate with you as you watch your weight, pain, and fatigue melt away.

Look for diet partners all around you—what about your church or your book club? Or maybe even consider doing a challenge at your workplace. We have seen people pool money for a prize for the person who loses the most weight and has the most drastic change in health.

2. LEAN ON US

We have created a support group and provided additional materials on our website, WholeLifeNutrition.net, to make your life easier. Even if you don't manage to form your own tribe at home, we would love to have you as part of ours! Visit our site and see all the resources we have to offer.

3. SET YOUR MIND-SET

To help you get off on the right foot, I want you to start thinking positive thoughts about your experience to come. But what if you can't jump right into that mental space? It helps to stop for a minute and perform a quick thought exercise.

Take a moment and contemplate your worst thoughts about your upcoming Elimination Diet experience. It could be things like, "This is going to be impossible!" or "There is no way I can go 24 hours without coffee or cheese!" Get them all out on the table. Then, just as easily, I want you to spout out the opposite: "This is totally doable!" and "Cheese and chocolate are highly overrated. I can do this!"

Such simple and playful shifts in your thinking can be life changing. By taking control of your thoughts, you are taking control of your attitude. Practice your positive thoughts—say them out loud, write them in your journal, or tell your friends and family. And soon enough you may find that you have the attitude that, no matter what happens, it's all good! Especially when you know that these challenges will be well worth it when you start to feel better.

4. DOCUMENT YOUR DIET DISCOVERIES

I want you to begin to think of yourself as a detective, searching for the pesky food suspects that are behind your symptoms and suffering. Begin to carry a journal around with you everywhere you go. Write down all the foods you eat and beverages you drink, and then if you notice any symptoms at all, write them down in the journal. Does this idea seem a little tedious to you? Trust me. It is a lot less tedious than missing what foods are causing you suffering. And if you consider this an exciting experiment, the journaling becomes really fun. Some of your reactions to foods can be pretty sneaky. You could get just a little sleepy or gassy after eating certain foods or you may get a flushing of your skin and have your sinuses start to drip a little. These may seem like normal occurrences that are unrelated to any foods...until you journal about them and begin to see connections to what you're eating.

Once you begin to document your symptoms, you will likely see that they occur within a certain time frame after eating a particular food. Lose the food and you will likely lose the symptoms. Without journaling, you will probably never clearly identify these connections.

The lessons you can learn from your journal should not be underestimated. I have looked back at my journals from years ago and have been able to figure out what's contributing to my current symptoms of fatigue, foggy thinking, joint pain, bowel problems, rashes, cranky moods, and more.

I know now the questions to ask myself: Is it the fructose in the green apples? Is it the cross contamination of gluten in the granola I just bought? If you know the symptoms that are associated with a particular food (because you wrote about it in your journal), you can quickly find the culprit and stop the symptoms. You, too, will discover the right questions to ask yourself and identify the answers once you complete the Elimination Diet.

It is a great idea to start journaling as soon as you can. I personally will carry around two journals when I am doing the Elimination Diet (I follow the program periodically when I feel it's time for a reset). One will be the full-size journal that gets the majority of the notes, and the other will be a pocket-size journal that goes everywhere with me—including, but not limited to, the bathroom. How else do you think I am going to track my bowel movements?

You can also use our Elimination Diet Journal to record your diet and any symptoms you may experience. You'll see a sample version here; for a free printable PDF, visit our website at WholeLifeNutrition.net.

ELIMINATION DIET JOURNAL
SAMPLE PAGE

Your journal will become an incredible tool as you go through the elimination diet program. Keep your journal with you at all times.

The day you begin the diet, take note of what you ate for breakfast, lunch, dinner, and snacks. Also, be sure to include how much water you drank throughout the day. Did you know that dehydration can produce symptoms similar to a food sensitivity? Be sure to drink enough water to hydrate your body, and to assist in detoxification.

There is a column next to what you ate where you can add any symptoms you experience after eating that particular meal. Be sure to fill this in within a few hours after eating. You might add words like: bloated, gassy, nauseous; or you might add things like calm gut, feeling energized, and clear mind. Take note of other symptoms like headaches, brain fog, achy muscles, pressure in sinuses, postnasal drip, bad breath, body odor, or heart palpitations.

DAY____7____   DATE: _____3/22/14_____
PHASE: 1 ② 3 _____   Challenge Food (Phase 3 only) _____n/a_____

BREAKFAST TIME: 7:30	16 ounces water, then 3½ cups Very Berry Chia Smoothie	tons of energy, BM: soft, formed
LUNCH TIME: 12:00	Turkey Hash, baby lettuce salad, Green Goddess Dressing	feeling good, happy, light, energetic
SNACK TIME: 2:30	16 ounces water, 1 large Granny Smith apple	bloated 30 minutes after eating
DINNER TIME: 7:00	Mint-ginger tea, cooked quinoa, roasted chicken, steamed asparagus, sweet potato mash	still feeling gassy, bloated, mood is a little cranky
BEVERAGES	Drank close to 80 ounces of water all day, 2 cups of homemade mint-ginger tea	
ADDITIONAL NOTES: ■ bowel movements ■ hours of sleep ■ infections ■ social occasions ■ menstrual cycle ■ stressful events	slept deeply for 7 hours, day 26 of menstrual cycle, feeling pretty good overall, clear mind	

5. LIFE IS TOUGH: TRY TAKING A BATH!

Life is stressful enough without completely turning your diet upside down. That's why as you prepare for and do the Elimination Diet, it will be especially important for you to set aside a little time every day to relax and let that stress dissipate.

One of the best ways to accomplish this is to take a bath, but not just any bath: an Epsom salt bath. Enjoying a nice hot bath with two cups of Epsom salts will do wonders to calm your body and your mind. Epsom salts contain magnesium and sulfate, which will work to settle your racing thoughts, allow your muscles to release, and give your liver a chance to efficiently metabolize both foods and toxins.

When you are fully at ease, your body will switch from a "fight or flight" mode to a state of "rest and digest." This will allow your intestines to calm and for cellular recovery to take place. While making drastic dietary changes, these baths will give you a break from extra stress and boost detoxification, making your Elimination Diet adventure much more enjoyable.

Epsom salt baths can also relieve many other sources of discomfort, such as:

- Anxiety
- Fatigue
- Flu-like symptoms
- Headaches
- Insomnia
- Joint pain
- Muscle tension/spasms
- Racing thoughts

If your skin tends to be dry, be sure to add ¼ cup of baking soda to the bath as well. Your skin will come out feeling silky and smooth.

6. GET SOME SUN

The warmth of the sun on your skin can calm down your entire nervous system, while the brightness of the sunlight can change neurotransmitters in your brain to improve your mood. Those reasons alone are enough to soak up some sun, but there's more.

When sunlight of a particular strength strikes your bare skin, it can change the shape of a cholesterol molecule under the surface, forming vitamin D3. This substance will then travel to your liver where it becomes something called 25-hydroxy vitamin D—this is what your doctor keeps track of to see if you have enough vitamin D for optimal health.

Vitamin D is important to so many critical functions in the body. In fact, if you could only track just *one* nutrient to make sure you had enough of it, vitamin D would be high on my short list.

What's the ideal level for vitamin D? There is currently some debate around what's considered to be "adequate." Many physicians will say that somewhere between 25 and 32 ng/ml is enough, but after reading thousands of articles on the subject, listening to world renowned experts debate the topic, and lecturing across North America about this vitamin, I am leaning toward 40 to 60 ng/ml. At these higher levels, I have seen that bone density, immune function, and disease prevention are optimized.

Here are some of the common improvements I see with optimal vitamin D levels:

- Better energy
- Calmer intestinal tracts
- Improved thyroid function
- Increased bone density
- Joint pain improvement
- Less back and neck pain
- More optimistic mood
- Skin conditions clearing up

Next time you're at the doctor, ask for a 25-hydroxy vitamin D test. Or you could go to GrassrootsHealth.net and order your own finger-stick test. Their website also offers a downloadable chart that will help you determine what daily dose you may need in order to maintain their recommended 40 to 60 ng/ml level.

Because adequate vitamin D is extremely difficult to attain through diet, responsible sun exposure or supplementation is highly recommended. Responsible dosing from the sun is achieved by exposing your skin to sun for the necessary time to get a light pinking or darkening to your skin without burning. This is often referred to as a minimal erythemal dose or MED. In fair-skinned individuals this may be achieved in 15 to 20 minutes; in a person with olive-toned skin it may take 30 to 45 minutes; and in people who are dark skinned it may take 120 minutes or more. The more skin exposed, the better.

Based on the fact that 100 percent of our skin can get us around 10,000 IUs of vitamin D, we know that 6 percent of our skin exposed (our hands, neck, and face) will only get us around 600 IUs of vitamin D. Research indicates that an adult needs approximately 3,500 IUs per day, so aim to expose 35 percent of your body during your sun breaks.

FOOD FOR THOUGHT

If you would like a more accurate and convenient way to determine your needs, you can also use a phone application like D-minder.

Sunscreen application will inhibit the formation of vitamin D, so wait until after your MED is reached before you apply. Even low SPFs will prevent the vitamin D boost: an SPF of 8 will reduce the vitamin D conversion in your skin by 92.5 percent, and an SPF of 15 will reduce it by 98 percent.

In the United States, people who live above the 35th parallel will not be able to get adequate vitamin D from the sun from late fall to early spring. If you were to draw an imaginary line from west to east through Bakersfield, California, Oklahoma City, Oklahoma, and Raleigh, North Carolina, this would mark the 35th parallel. If you live in areas above this line, it's likely you will need to take a vitamin D supplement to maintain healthy levels.

People who have a history of skin cancer may want to limit their exposure to sun as well and rely on supplementation.

See Supplements to Support the Elimination Diet on page 107 for how to get enough vitamin D when natural sunlight isn't available to you or is not recommended.

7. HAVE SOME SOUP

Grandma was right. Everyone feels better after a good bowl of soup. All of the miraculous plant compounds from the herbs, vegetables, and spices have time to steep into every warm spoonful of goodness. If you choose to make chicken soup or bone broth, the gut-healing proline and glycine amino acids will help to soothe and repair any damage, while also supporting optimal muscle tone and detoxification. Because soups are cooked thoroughly, they are easy to digest and often tolerated by people with upset intestinal tracts.

Plus, soups are easy! You just chop up the ingredients, throw them in a pot, and set a timer. Done. Then you have meals for days, if not weeks. If you make a big batch, it's easy to prep the leftovers for storage. Here's how we do it at our house:

- Pour cooked soup into clean mason jars to cool, leaving a few inches at the top so the soup can expand.
- Place the jars in the freezer (with the lids still off to leave room for expansion and prevent the jars from cracking) and wait until the soup freezes (usually overnight).
- Put the lids on the next day and leave the soup in the freezer for a rainy or busy day.

Having your freezer stocked with some soups or broths can make your life and your Elimination Diet a breeze. Any time you are hungry, just run to the freezer, thaw out a jar of soup, drop it into a pot, and enjoy. Add some fresh vegetables or meats and you have a delicious, nutritious, lightning-fast meal.

8. MAKE SMOOTHIES

What's easier to make than a soup? A smoothie! During the Elimination Diet, it is a great idea to have your freezer stocked with lots of organic fruits, and your fridge loaded with green leafy vegetables. Adding in some hemp seeds and/or ground chia seeds (or whole seeds if you have a high-powered blender like a Vitamix) can help to tide you over for a while. There really is nothing simpler than grabbing items, throwing them in a blender, and turning it on.

Does making a fruit-and-vegetable smoothie sound weird to you? It's okay if it does, especially if you're not used to eating many fresh fruits and vegetables in your regular diet. One of the great benefits of the Elimination Diet is that it helps reset your taste buds so that you start to crave fresh, whole foods instead of artificial, processed foods. So before too long on the Elimination Diet, you'll come to discover how delicious a fresh smoothie like this can be! You really can't go wrong by putting a bunch of healthy ingredients into a blender and giving it a spin.

Here are the staples that make up our organic smoothies:

Organic Fresh or Frozen Fruits:
Apples
Bananas*
Blueberries (wild are great, too)*
Cherries
Mangoes
Papaya*
Pears
Pineapple*
Raspberries*
Strawberries*

*Indicates fruits that are lower in fermentable carbohydrates (aka fermentable oligosaccharides, disaccharides, monosaccharides, and polylols or FOD-MAPs; see page 180 for more on a low-FODMAP diet). Fruits and other foods high in these fermentable carbohydrates are readily eaten (fermented) by intestinal bacteria and this can lead to bloating, gas, and irritable bowel symptoms.

Organic Fresh Greens and Vegetables:
Avocados
Collards
Cucumbers
Ginger
Kales (black/lacinato, red, Siberian)
Napa cabbage

Organic Seeds:

Ground chia seeds (or whole seeds if you have a high-powered blender
   like the Vitamix or BlendTec)
Hemp seeds

Not only are smoothies easy, but when made with the right ingredients, they can provide an incredible number of health benefits. Now, I'm not talking about the typical smoothie you get at a chain smoothie shop, which can be overloaded with sugar and other reactive ingredients like dairy and artificial flavors. I'm talking about healing and satisfying smoothies that are made from only fresh, replenishing whole foods.

For example: If you were to toss kale, ginger, blueberries, pineapple, ground chia seeds, and water into a blender, you would have one of the most potent antioxidant drinks you could dream up.

Kale contains sulforaphane, a potent detoxification and antioxidant chemical.

Ginger is an anti-inflammatory powerhouse thanks to its gingerols, which have shown to benefit 75 percent of joint-pain sufferers and 100 percent of muscle-pain sufferers.

Blueberries are rich in anthocyanadins, which are powerful antioxidants that protect brain function.

Pineapple is chock-full of vitamin C—1 cup of this tropical fruit exceeds your daily requirement.

Chia seeds are a fantastic source of fiber and omega-3 fatty acids: Less than an ounce of ground chia seeds a day has been shown to increase the anti-inflammatory omega-3 fatty acid EPA by 39 percent.

See how easy (and tasty) it can be to drink to your great health? And that is just the tip of the iceberg. I had a gentleman come into my office who wanted to lose weight. He was not willing to cut out gluten, dairy, or any other foods to reach his goals. The *only* thing he was willing to commit to was to drinking a green smoothie every morning. After twenty-eight days, he had lost 15 pounds!

Common improvements I see with green smoothies:

- Better mood
- Glowing skin

- Improved energy
- Weight loss

Be sure to check out all the great smoothie recipes in chapter 11.

9. GROW YOUR OWN KITCHEN GARDEN

Growing things is fun. Really fun. And in the case of growing your own broccoli sprouts, it may be one of the healthiest things you can do for yourself.

In 1992, a team of scientists from Johns Hopkins University searched the globe for miraculous compounds that could protect our cells from cancer. And they found them in a common group of vegetables many of us eat called cruciferous vegetables. These are:

- Arugula
- Broccoli
- Brussels sprouts
- Cabbage
- Cauliflower
- Kale
- Radishes
- Watercress

The way they protect us is fascinating. These vegetables contain a chemical called sulforaphane that allows our genes to make more antioxidant and detoxification proteins. Regular antioxidants like vitamin C fight free radicals directly and protect us for approximately 6 hours after we are exposed to damaging chemicals. But sulforaphane is an even more powerful protector— it ramps up the ability of each and every one of our cells to secrete hundreds of antioxidant and detoxification chemicals for more than 72 hours.

Research has shown that when people eat foods high in sulforaphane, they are protected from air pollution, heavy metals, pesticides, and many other compounds. And what food is particularly high in sulforaphane? Broccoli sprouts. Broccoli sprouts are shown to have more than *20 times* the amount of sulforaphane as regular broccoli. (See Tom's TEDx talk, "Broccoli—The DNA Whisperer" at http://tedxtalks.ted.com/video/Broccoli-The-DNA-Whisperer-Tom.)

So get sprouting! Check out the video on our website and the recipe on page 301. Then, buy all the supplies you need and jump right in. I advise all my clients to start sprouting broccoli seeds, and most of them have grown addicted to the fun and healthy process. Not only do they experience noticeable shifts in their health when they eat the sprouts, but they seem to adore the process of watching their little plants grow on their kitchen counters. Kids love to be included in the process, too.

10. HAVE A BUBBLING KITCHEN

Beneficial bacteria (aka probiotics) are our friends. Cultures across the globe have known this for millennia, which is why you'll continue to find what I call "bubbling foods" in their kitchens. Bubbling foods are fermented foods, such as sauerkraut, kefir, yogurt, pickles, and fermented meats. When you enjoy them, you introduce incredible beneficial bacteria into your diet. It's a time-tested tradition worth following.

I once had a young man come up to me and thank me for the cultured vegetable information that we share on our blog and in our books. He told me that it saved him from months of severe intestinal pain. After a hernia surgery left him with an infection, his doctors put him on a course of antibiotics. Soon after, he started having terrible bloating, gas, cramping, and erratic bowel movements, all of which continued for months.

It wasn't until he started eating sauerkraut that he began to feel better. After two weeks of regular consumption, his symptoms were nearly gone. A few months later, he said, "I was a new man!" And all just from eating sauerkraut.

The beneficial bacteria found in fermented foods can create a profound change in the gut environment. They help reestablish balance, which can relieve digestive distress; ward off infection and boost your immune system; and increase energy by replenishing several important nutrients, including many B vitamins.

The easiest way to start your adventure into fermented foods is with lacto-fermented vegetables. The process of making them is almost as simple as making a smoothie. You just chop up some veggies, put them in a jar with salt water, put the lid on, and wait. About a week later, they are ready to enjoy. Just enter "lacto-fermented vegetables" into the search bar on our NourishingMeals.com blog for an instructional video. (Turn to page 297 in chapter 11 for some easy recipes to try.)

You can eat these vegetables on their own—they're great as snacks and sides. But they're also excellent as a condiment. Several of my clients like to use cultured vegetables this way to add flare to otherwise bland dishes. Personally, I've found that adding sauerkraut or lacto-fermented cauliflower to some steamed or roasted kabocha squash can really kick up the flavor; the mixture of tangy and sweet is amazing. And I have yet to find any meal that does not go well with a side of fermented green beans. Something magical happens to green beans when they are fermented for a few weeks. Even our kids eat them like candy, as our jars quickly disappear from our countertop.

Long story short . . . fermented and bubbling foods taste great, are fun and easy to make, and will assist you in feeling great.

SUPPLEMENTS TO SUPPORT THE ELIMINATION DIET

There are a handful of supplements that I like to recommend for most people before and during the Elimination Diet. The supplements will support you on this program in a variety of ways.

It's important to note that this information should not serve as a replacement for advice from your own health-care practitioner. I recommend searching for a practitioner trained in Functional Medicine. You can find out if there are any in your area by going to the website of the Institute of Functional Medicine (functionalmedicine.org). Click on "Find a Practitioner" at the top of the website and enter the required information.

For specific brand recommendations, you can see the resource guide in the back of this book, or visit us at WholeLifeNutrition.net for more information.

1. **Multivitamin:** Many people are not meeting their daily requirement for essential nutrients. This is due in part to our mineral-depleted soils and our polluted environment. But it's also a product of dysfunctional intestinal tracts (which don't properly absorb nutrients) and a poor diet. These factors have combined to make malnutrition quite common these days.

The simple addition of a high-quality, easily absorbed multivitamin can be a huge step in the right direction toward recovering your health. In my own clients, I've seen the right type of multivitamin produce drastic improvements.

2. **Vitamin D:** If your vitamin D levels are not in the 40 to 60 ng/ml range, and you are not getting adequate sun exposure, supplementation with vitamin D3 may be called for. (See also Get Some Sun on page 99.) The Grassrootshealth.com website chart will give you an indication as to how much vitamin D you may need to supplement. Be sure to take some vitamin K2 along with your D3 as they work together to put calcium where it needs to go. (See the Resources section on page 303 for supplement recommendations.)

3. **Essential Fatty Acids:** A purified fish oil product can be very beneficial for people who are not consuming regular amounts of fish. Many people will find benefits from taking a combination of 1.5 to 3 grams of EPA and DHA a day. It is important that you choose a high-quality product as there is potential for contamination of fish oils with heavy metals, PCBs, and other ocean pollutants.

4. **Magnesium:** Magnesium is the most important mineral in the human body, as it is a cofactor for more than 300 enzymes. It helps regulate blood sugar and blood pressure, and maintains relaxation in your muscles. Magnesium also has the honored task of carrying something called adenosine triphosphate (ATP) around. This is your cellular currency, or what your body relies on to produce energy. When things go wrong with ATP, your cells have trouble functioning. As a result of this dysfunction, you can feel fatigued, agitated, and unmotivated (see the sidebar on page 109 for other magnesium deficiency symptoms).

Your body also requires adequate levels of magnesium for digestion and detoxification, and to help regulate bowel movements. Irregular bowel movements, especially constipation, can cause the walls of the lower intestines to reabsorb the toxins your body has worked so hard to clear out. This is one of the reasons you feel so lousy after you have been constipated for a few days.

One of the safest ways of encouraging bowels to move again is the supplementation of magnesium. Most people find that their bowel movements are easier after supplementing with 400 to 600 mg of magnesium citrate. Some health-care practitioners will recommend upward of 1,000 mg if a client is suffering from constipation. Please be aware that this may cause a bowel movement that may occur within 6 hours' time (i.e., you will not want to be far from a toilet). Other forms of magnesium, such as magnesium glycinate or taurate, tend to be milder on your intestines and may be more appropriate for people who are not suffering from constipation.

As a maintenance dose, many Functional Medicine practitioners will recommend daily supplementation of 200 to 400 mg to assure adequate magnesium status. Frequent Epsom salt baths can assist you in meeting your magnesium requirements as well. Check with your health-care practitioner to determine the magnesium supplementation that's best for you.

ARE YOU DEFICIENT IN MAGNESIUM?

If you have a magnesium deficiency, you could experience any of the following symptoms:

- Never really feel awake, always tired
- Startled by loud noises
- Often anxious and can't seem to calm down
- Have racing thoughts
- Muscle cramping (neck, back, and jaw pain are common)
- Trouble falling asleep and staying asleep
- Twitching in the legs or feet
- Numbness and tingling in legs, feet, and toes
- Loss of appetite
- Racing or abnormal heartbeat
- Carb cravings and blood sugar regulation issues (insulin resistance)

5. **Activated Charcoal:** When acute toxic chemical exposure lands someone in the emergency room, activated charcoal will often be used to treat them. This is because activated charcoal binds to toxins in the intestinal tract and helps excrete them from the body.

When you are making big dietary changes, you may free up toxins that have been locked into the cells and tissues of your body. This sort of toxic release can produce symptoms of lethargy, joint pain, and headaches. It is possible for these detox symptoms to set in while you are doing the

Elimination Diet. Having a bottle of activated charcoal around may assist you in neutralizing these toxins, which will improve or lessen the time you have to tolerate any such symptoms. Follow the recommendations on the product you choose.

6. **Sulfur to the Rescue!** When you are exposed to a toxin, it will almost always make its way to the liver. It is here that most "detoxification" takes place. If the body is going through a process that may bring about a great purging of toxins—such as the Elimination Diet—the liver can use all the help it can get. That's where sulfur comes in.

Sulfur-based compounds are used in the body to neutralize toxins. These compounds have names like sulfate, glutathione, taurine, and methionine. Here are the actions you can take to optimize detoxification:

- **Make sure you're eating broccoli sprouts.** Broccoli sprouts are one of the most potent detoxification-supporting substances on the planet. Not only do they ramp up our cells' ability to produce detoxification enzymes, but they also increase your production of glutathione, an extremely important toxin neutralizer.
- **Eat sulfur-rich foods.** These include broccoli, Brussels sprouts, garlic, radishes, arugula, and onions.
- **Take Epsom salt baths.** There are two main ingredients in these salts: magnesium and the sulfur salt called sulfate. This sulfur source can pass readily into your body through your skin and increase your sulfur stores.
- **Take a toxin-removing supplement.** There are supplements designed to supply the ingredients necessary for excreting reactive toxins. The best product that's backed by research is called n-acetyl cysteine or NAC. Cysteine is the most important component of a master antioxidant in the body called glutathione. When you have more glutathione, you are better able to detox. When you have more NAC, you have more glutathione. Another product I recommend is called Solvent Remover, made by Thorne Research. It contains n-acetyl cysteine, glycine, l-glutamine, lipoic acid, and taurine. You can find this on our website and from Functional Medicine practitioners. There are many other products that work beautifully for detoxification, and I recommend you discuss these with your health-care provider.

7. **Probiotics:** We've talked about a great way for you to get beneficial bacteria from fermented foods (see page 106), but you can also get them from probiotic supplements. I'm sure you've heard about probiotics, and you've probably wondered if they live up to the hype.

Here's the truth: It depends on too many factors to know if they will work for your specific condition or symptoms. As it stands, there are some bifidobacteria and lactobacilli strains that have great research behind them. Names like Culturelle, Phillips' Colon Health, VSL-3, and Florastor are all known to have great results on conditions such as traveler's diarrhea, *C. difficile* infections, and ulcerative colitis. I highly recommend you seek out a practitioner trained in Functional Medicine to help you navigate this ever-growing field of information.

Here's what to look for when choosing a probiotic:

- **Look for a reputable brand of supplements.** Probiotics are living organisms. If they aren't treated well (e.g., they're exposed to high heat or excessive moisture) or fed properly, or they are combined with competitive organisms, you will be buying a bottle of dead microbes. Make sure you have validated the brand you are choosing via a skilled practitioner who is familiar with probiotics.
- **Check the bottle.** When you are looking at the amount of probiotics in the bottle, see if the colony-forming units (CFUs) are listed as "at time of bottling" or "at time of expiration." If the probiotics say "at time of bottling," then you need to pay attention to the dates on the bottle. The fresher the bottle, the better your results are likely to be. So look through the shelf and find the product with the most recent date.
- **Take a diverse selection of organisms.** Research continues to prove how important it is to have a wide range of organisms in your intestinal tract. Each organism has a distinct job, and it is difficult to determine which one will benefit you the most without proper lab analysis. In the near future, you will be able to get a sample of your microbiome from different parts of your intestinal tract taken and get a specific recommendation for the specific condition you are suffering from. Until that happens, try a wide variety of probiotics with the guidance of your health-care practitioner to see which products benefit your symptoms the most.

8. **Berberine:** For people who have intestinal imbalances like SIBO, irritable bowel, or inflammatory bowel, I will often recommend a trial with berberine extract. The bright yellow bitter alkaloids found in berberine have been used for centuries for balancing out intestinal microbes. Recent science is showing their efficacy in regulating blood sugar and body weight as well. The standard adult dosing varies between 300 and 1,500 mg of berberine per day.

9. **Meriva:** Many people who are suffering from arthritis, back pain, muscle aches and pains, irritated bowels, and other symptoms of inflammation resort to taking over-the-counter and/or prescription anti-inflammatories. Unfortunately, one of the primary side effects associated with these medications is intestinal damage. If recent science reveals that much of our inflammation originates in the gut, and the medications we're using to calm inflammation are harming the gut, doesn't this seem a bit counterproductive?

Thankfully, there are better, natural options making their way to the marketplace. A 2013 article in the *Journal of Pain Research* showed that a plant extract supplement derived from turmeric known as Meriva is as effective at lowering pain as acetaminophen (Tylenol). And it doesn't just lower pain, it also lowers inflammation. An article from *Alternative Medicine Review* in 2010 demonstrated the power of Meriva to significantly lower markers of inflammation like high-sensitivity C-reactive protein (hs-CRP) in patients with arthritis.

Meriva also has a history of showing no intestinal upset or liver damage. In fact, it shows the exact opposite. Studies on inflammatory bowel disease and fatty liver disease demonstrate that the plant chemicals found in Meriva can be quite protective of both the intestines and the liver. In short, Meriva lowers pain and inflammation without the adverse side effects of commonly used medication. There are side effects, however. Good ones. Meriva and other turmeric-based supplements are being used to prevent cancers as well.

The maintenance dosing of Meriva as an anti-inflammatory is recommended to be 1 to 1.5 grams (1,000 to 1,500 mg) per day. The article on pain reduction showed dosing of 4 grams (4,000 mg).

10. **Digestive Enzymes:** If you have suffered from terrible gas, bloating, multiple loose bowel movements per day, or urgent bowel movements that float, or you see lots of undigested food in your stool, the addition of digestive enzymes may change your life.

In general, animal-based enzymes with pig-derived pancreatic enzymes and ox bile are excellent for people with sluggish digestion. However, during the Elimination Diet, I recommend plant-based enzymes instead, since many of the animal-derived enzymes will have both beef- and pork-sourced ingredients in them. I typically recommend taking digestive enzymes with each meal before beginning the Elimination Diet and through the duration of the diet. If someone has a known sensitivity to aspergillus, a microbe used in the making of some plant enzymes, they may need to be avoided altogether.

Follow the specific directions on the bottle of the product you buy. If you are suffering from terrible bloating, nausea, cramping, and erratic bowel movements, you may need to take more enzymes than are recommended on the label, but be sure to consult a Functional Medicine–trained practitioner before doing so.

If you have floating and urgent stools, choose a product designed for fat digestion that has a significant amount of lipase. See the Resource section in the back of this book for recommended brand names.

Digestive enzymes can help:

- Control small intestinal bacterial overgrowth (SIBO)
- Increase your ability to get nutrients from your food, allowing for more energy and overall vitality
- Lessen diarrhea and constipation
- Relieve gas, nausea, and bloating

I want you to keep in mind that all these steps and supplements are intended to provide you with the maximum support as you prepare for and follow the Elimination Diet. They are not essential, but in many cases will provide physical and mental boosts that will only make the process easier for you. You will find resources for these supplements on our supplementation page at WholeLifeNutrition.net. Implement what you can, take note of what proves successful for you, and modify or remove what doesn't. Remember this is just the start of your journey toward creating a customized diet that will promote complete healing.

6

THE ELIMINATION KITCHEN

Now comes the fun part! One of the best perks of the Elimination Diet is all of the delicious food you'll be eating to promote healing and boost your overall health and wellness. Most people find that the Elimination Diet inspires them to eat a more varied diet, full of tasty new seasonings and flavors, and this culinary adventure starts before you take your first step in phase one of the program: It starts by preparing your kitchen for this exciting adventure to better health, one bite at a time.

Before you begin the Elimination Diet, set yourself up for success by making sure you have the proper equipment and food stocked in your kitchen. It's important that you start to think of your kitchen as your epicenter of wellness—from this space, you will create the meals that repair your gut, restart your metabolism, and remove your symptoms. Set it up with the knowledge that a little upfront effort will generate nothing short of life-changing results.

You will be more successful on the Elimination Diet if you take the time to prepare instead of jumping right in.

UPGRADE YOUR KITCHEN TOOLS

What you use in your kitchen matters. You want the materials and surfaces you use for cooking to be free of contaminants and chemicals. In general, you should aim to have more tools that are made from glass, wood, or stainless steel and less of those made from plastics and synthetic materials. Before you begin the Elimination Diet, try to:

Purge your kitchen of nonstick pots, pans, and bakeware. There are chemicals in nonstick surfaces that have been linked to thyroid disorders, infertility, developmental disorders, and more.

Remove plastic storage containers. Replace these with glass or stainless steel for storing food. When exposed to heat, freezing, and acids (like those found in vinegar, lemon, or tomato products), compounds in plastics can leach into your food and shift your immune cells to be more allergenic, leading to an increase in asthma, eczema, and food reactions. As discussed in chapter 4, BPA and phthalates in plastics also disrupt blood sugar metabolism, leading to an increased risk for type 2 diabetes and obesity.

You will also want to invest in some pieces of kitchen equipment that will be invaluable assets to you during the Elimination Diet. These items will help you make the recipes in chapter 11, which have been written exclusively to help nourish and heal your body. It's likely you have some of these items already, but be sure to pick up the ones you don't:

- Food processor
- High-powered blender and/or juicer
- Stainless steel immersion blender
- Small wooden citrus juicer
- Garlic press
- Stainless steel grater
- New wooden cutting boards that have not been contaminated with gluten
- High-quality sharp knives
- Measuring cups and spoons
- Large bamboo or wooden spoons not contaminated with gluten
- Stainless steel spatulas
- Large stainless steel colander
- Fine-mesh strainer
- 8-quart stainless steel pot with lid
- 2-quart heavy-bottomed stainless steel pot with lid
- Deep 11- to 12-inch stainless steel or cast-iron skillet
- 10-inch cast-iron skillet
- 8-inch cast-iron tortilla press
- Widemouthed quart jars
- Glass and stainless steel food storage containers in different sizes

PREPARE TO GET THE MOST OUT OF YOUR MEALS

You will be more successful on the Elimination Diet if you utilize leftovers. The more you prepare fresh meals for yourself, the greater your motivation will be to use every last bit of delicious nourishment you've cooked. And keep in mind that just because you had a food one way for dinner doesn't mean you have to eat it the same way for lunch the next day. Here are some of our favorite leftover meals:

- Pair roasted chicken with leftover baked squash and some fresh salad greens; place it all in a stainless steel to-go container for a simple, tasty meal.
- Add cooked beans and steamed vegetables to leftover quinoa and toss with your favorite Elimination Diet salad dressing (see pages 271 to 276 for dressings).
- Mix leftover salmon with steamed kale, roasted carrots, and sliced avocado for a quick and healthy meal.
- Heat up leftover chicken vegetable soup—or any of the soups included in chapter 11—and place it in a stainless steel thermos to go. Soups are perfect for when you're busy and tight on time, and they're full of nourishment.

To get the most from your foods, be sure to store items in airtight containers. Use these guidelines to determine how long foods can safely be consumed:

- Cooked meat will last in the refrigerator for up to 5 days.
- Cooked salmon will last in the refrigerator for up to 3 days.

- Cooked vegetables will last in the refrigerator for up to 1 week.
- Cooked whole grains and beans will last in the refrigerator for 5 to 7 days.

HOW TO SHOP FOR HERBS AND SPICES

Herbs and spices begin as fresh, whole ingredients that are ground down for use in cooking. It's important to know that the starting ingredients are of high quality. Look for spices that are organic and gluten-free. You can also try growing your own herbs. Growing a planter box garden of oregano, thyme, mint, sage, chives, and rosemary is much easier and more rewarding than you could ever imagine. Throw some lavender in there so you can get a whiff of its calming fragrance while you are harvesting your bounty.

STOCKING YOUR ELIMINATION DIET KITCHEN

When we buy food, we are buying the most important commodity in our lives. Why's it so important? Because from the cellular to the surface level, your food choices form who you are. You want great skin and hair, a sharp mind, clear eyes, and a calm gut? Eat nutrient-dense, whole foods. It's that simple.

Think of shopping as a skill. Sure, you know how to do it, but it's something at which you can improve. Here's how to be a smart shopper:

THE EVOLVING MARKETPLACE

Many local food stores recognize the growing interest in gluten- and dairy-free diets and diets free of other reactive foods. Some stores offer free tours and cooking and other educational classes on how to live a healthier life. Check out the local health food stores in your area to take advantage of what they have to offer.

1. **Find a store that is much smarter about organics and fresh foods than you are.** Ask your local co-op or health food store if they have a nutritionist on staff who could point out some of the nutritional highlights of their store.

2. **Locate the nearest farmers' market and visit soon and often.** There is no better meal than one that is prepared with super-fresh, organic produce that has been picked that day. Carrots and peas will taste sweet enough to have for dessert, and berries and greens will give you an antioxidant buzz. You can also meet the most down-to-earth and educated people at these markets. Many will have a solid background on sustainable agriculture and some will even give fabulous cooking tips on preparing the produce you're purchasing from them. It is here that you will often find out about local, sustainably raised animal products as well.

3. **Seek out a local butcher or meat supplier who works with organic, pasture-finished animals.** Not only will you get the freshest meats around, you are likely to support a farming system that will preserve life on this planet for many generations to come.

GROCERY GUIDANCE

Visit our website, **WholeLifeNutrition.net**, to download our handy grocery shopping guide for Stocking Your Elimination Diet Kitchen.

At the Store

Don't stress—we've got your grocery list covered. Here are all the foods you need to stock up on for the Elimination Diet.

The Elimination Diet Shopping List

(See WholeLifeNutrition.net for a PDF version of this list)

WHOLE GRAINS:
Amaranth flour
Brown rice (preferably organic and sprouted)
Brown rice flour (preferably organic and sprouted)
Quinoa

Quinoa flour
White jasmine rice
Wild rice

LEGUMES:
Adzuki beans
Black beans
Garbanzo bean flour (preferably
    organic and sprouted)
Garbanzo beans
Lima beans
Mung beans
Pinto and pink beans
White beans

MEATS AND FISH:
Anchovies
Black cod
Chicken: whole chicken,
    chicken breasts, and thighs
    (organic)
Lamb: ground lamb (organic)
Turkey: Bone-in turkey breasts
    or thighs, ground turkey
    (organic)
Wild salmon
Wild scallops

FRUITS:
Apples
Apricots: fresh or dried with no
    added preservatives
Bananas
Berries: blueberries,
    blackberries, raspberries,
    strawberries
Cherries

Dates: dried or fresh with no
    preservatives or additives
Figs: dried or fresh
Grapes
Melons
Nectarines and peaches
Papayas
Pears
Pineapple
Plums
Pomegranates

VEGETABLES:
Artichokes
Asparagus
Avocados
Beets
Bok choy
Broccoli
Brussels sprouts
Cabbage
Carrots
Cauliflower
Celeriac
Celery
Chard
Cilantro (coriander)
Collard greens
Cucumber
Fennel
Garlic
Ginger
Jerusalem artichokes (sunchokes)
Kale
Lettuce (all varieties except
    iceberg)

Mizuna

Mushrooms

Mustard greens

Onions

Parsley

Parsnip

Peas: sugar snap, snow, frozen,
and dried split

Pickles: homemade without
peppers

Pumpkin

Rutabaga

Spinach

String beans

Sweet potatoes

Turnips

Watercress

Winter squash: all varieties

Yams

Zucchini

SEA VEGETABLES:

Arame

Dulse

Hijiki

Kombu

Nori

SEEDS AND BUTTERS:

Chia seeds: raw

Hemp seeds: raw

Pumpkin seed butter: raw

Pumpkin seeds: raw

Sunflower seeds: raw

OILS AND VINEGARS:

Extra-virgin olive oil

Raw organic apple cider vinegar

Raw organic coconut vinegar

Virgin coconut oil

SWEETENERS:

Coconut sugar

Pure maple syrup

Raw honey

HERBAL TEAS:

Astragalus

Burdock

Chamomile

Dandelion root

Ginger

Lemon balm

Licorice

Mint

Nettle

Rooibos

Rose

Slippery elm

Tulsi (holy basil)

Valerian

DRIED HERBS AND SPICES:

Bay leaves

Black peppercorns

Cardamom: ground

Cinnamon: ground and whole
sticks

Coriander: ground

Cumin: ground and whole seeds

Dill: dried

Ginger: ground

Nutmeg: ground

Oregano: dried

Thyme: dried
Turmeric: ground

OTHER INGREDIENTS:
Arrowroot powder (make sure it
    comes from a gluten-free facility)
Coconut aminos
Coconut milk (canned, organic)
Herbamare
Sea salt (such as Redmond Real
    Salt, Celtic sea salt, Himalayan
    pink salt)
Vanilla powder (raw organic)

PART III

Heal Yourself with the Elimination Diet

Our Elimination Diet program starts with a detoxification phase (phase 1) followed by a phase of balancing neutral foods (phase 2), and then ends with the reintroduction phase (phase 3), where you slowly add back in potentially reactive foods.

One general suggestion is to be strategic about when you schedule the diet—it's best not to do it during the holiday season. Holiday foods can be too tempting for you to successfully stay on the diet, and the higher stress levels during the season don't help, either. Of course, if your symptoms demand immediate attention and it happens to be the holiday season, do what's best for you. (It's just one snicker doodle; you'll live without it—even if it is your grandma's best recipe.)

All of the foods allowed in phases 1 and 2 of our Elimination Diet are neutral for most people. If at any point you don't feel well after eating one of the recipes, record your symptoms and foods consumed in your Elimination Diet Journal and remove the offending foods from your diet.

We have outlined some ways you can modify our diet based on additional food reactions, such as FODMAP sensitivities and starch maldigestion. Turn to page 180 for more information on how to further customize the Elimination Diet for these considerations.

A final note before you begin: If you follow the Elimination Diet as it's designed, you will be dedicating nearly two months to this program. It is a commitment. But I want you to put this in perspective to a lifetime of dealing with symptoms that *will only get worse* if you do nothing about them. Remember that uncontrolled, chronic inflammation in the body can lead to more than discomfort; it's linked to diabetes, heart disease, stroke, Alzheimer's, multiple sclerosis, thyroid issues, gallbladder disease, and arthritis, among other conditions and diseases.

By following the Elimination Diet, not only will you rid yourself of your symptoms, but you will also put an end to one of the most powerful disease initiators science has ever seen.

My ultimate goal is that you emerge, as so many of my clients have, on the other side of the Elimination Diet with a powerful, personalized way of eating that gives you the quality of life you deserve.

7

PHASE 1:

Detox—Days 1 and 2

Congratulations—just by reaching this point in the book, you've already made a clear commitment to your health and wellness. You are just a matter of days and meals away from feeling better than you have in years (or perhaps than you have ever felt), losing weight, healing your gut, reducing inflammation, and boosting overall health.

The Elimination Diet begins with a powerful detox phase that will jump-start your healing. Over the next two days, you will begin to calm your immune system and clear the gut. By eating to create a calm, clean intestinal slate, you will set yourself up to achieve the most accurate and amazing results during the next two phases of the diet. Think of these initial cleansing days as a rejuvenating trip to the spa for your digestive system.

During this phase, you will eat only fresh vegetable juices, green smoothies, and puréed cooked vegetables in homemade stock. A typical day might look like this:

- Green smoothie for breakfast
- Early lunch consisting of 1 quart of puréed vegetable soup
- 2 to 4 cups of fresh vegetable juice for an afternoon snack
- A bowl of puréed vegetable soup for dinner
- Herbal teas, purified water, and fresh coconut water enjoyed freely throughout the day

You should plan to eat this way for two days, at minimum. If you have a number of health issues, this phase can be extended for maximum benefit. For example, if you are experiencing gas, nausea, and bloating, or constipation and cramping, you can choose the low-FODMAP recipe options (see What is the FODMAP diet and do I need to follow it? on page 180 for more on the low-FODMAP diet) and extend the detox phase to four or more days. Because of the focused, limited selection of foods eaten during this phase, it should not extend beyond seven days—you need a more diverse and rich diet to support your health in the long term.

The foods and nutrients featured in this phase have been carefully selected to achieve three goals:

- Reduce inflammation in the intestines and immune cells
- Give the digestive tract a rest
- Provide a high amount of plant-based antioxidants

A full list of foods to eat and foods to avoid during phase 1 can be found beginning on page 133. Remember, the Elimination Diet isn't just about removing irritants; it's also about flooding your body with healing foods and nutrients that will repair the damage of years of eating reactive and irritating foods. Let me tell you a little more about the ingredients that will help cultivate a calm environment for your Elimination Diet experiment.

PHYTONUTRIENT-RICH VEGETABLES

Within the last few decades alone, scientists have found more than 40,000 different chemicals in plants that may be as important, if not more so, than the vitamins and minerals with which we are all familiar.

Plants interact with their environment just like we do, so as they are exposed to competitive weeds, insects, radiation from the sun, temperature changes, fungal infections, and other stressors, they produce defensive compounds known as phytochemicals. A couple of examples are carotenoids, which act as sunscreen for plants, and sulforaphane, which works as a natural pesticide. (You can check out my TEDx talk on sulforaphane online; visit our website, WholeLifeNutrition.net, for the link.) The very same compounds that protect these plants also protect us.

By eating lots of vegetables, we are trusting Mother Nature to provide us with the most health benefits possible. Every time you eat a vegetable-rich meal, you are gifting your cells with signals that will make them stronger and healthier. Food is not just flavor and macronutrients, but information— and vegetables deliver messages that promote optimal health and healing.

When foods like broccoli sprouts (more on these health-boosting sprouts on page 105) arrive in the body, they come carrying compounds such as sulforaphane, which literally turns on your cells' ability to produce powerful antioxidant and detoxification proteins.

Here's a little more on some of the other amazing compounds you'll find in vegetables:

Allicin: Organic compounds can help rid the intestinal tract of bad bacteria and naturally tamp down inflammatory chemicals in your body. You'll get more when you eat onions, leeks, and garlic. *Get them in this phase by trying*: Creamy Green Detox Soup (page 206).

Anthocyanins: Flavonoids are responsible for the bright and beautiful deep red and purple hues you'll find in many fruits and vegetables. Anthocyanins will help reduce inflammation and fight off free radicals, which are known to promote a cancer friendly environment. They are found in cranberries, plums, red cabbage, and cherries. *Get them in this phase by trying*: Red Cabbage and Berry Smoothie (page 193).

Carotenoids: Colorful pigments that produce oranges, yellows, and reds in fruits and vegetables. You probably know the carotenoid beta-carotene, which is found in carrots and is known for giving carrots their vibrant orange hue. Other foods such as broccoli and spinach have them, too, but you might not know it at first glance: The underlying color is hidden by the dominant greens created by chlorophyll. Carotenoids can reduce cell mutations that can lead to cancer and can disable inflammatory chemicals before they cause damage. *Get them in this phase by trying*: Carrot-Ginger-Shiitake Soup (page 207).

Indoles: Strong antioxidants that metabolize carcinogens, assist in DNA repair, and convert estrogen to a less cancer-promoting form. Indoles are found in cruciferous vegetables, such as cabbage, kale, broccoli, Brussels sprouts, and cauliflower. *Get them in this phase by trying*: Creamy Broccoli-Mushroom Soup (page 208).

PURIFIED WATER

Our bodies are composed primarily of water. Every cell functions better when it is well hydrated—you have more energy, better detoxification, and improved digestion when your cells have enough water in them. You are less likely to develop leaky gut when there is adequate fluid in your intestinal tract. Drinking 8 to 10 glasses of purified water every day will produce many noticeable benefits for you.

There's a reason I recommend purified water—several reasons, actually. Alarming amounts of antibiotics, pharmaceuticals, and industrial chemicals are ending up in our water supply, and standard city filtration is no longer sufficient to guarantee your safety. Additionally, many wells are also testing positive for chemical residues.

The good news is, reverse-osmosis water systems can provide an added level of protection. If there are high levels of lead, arsenic, or cadmium in the water, an added carbon block filter would also be a good idea.

If you don't have a filtration system at home, check your local grocery store. Many will have massive machines that filter water for you right in the store. All you have to do is bring in your glass containers and refill them there for a fraction of the cost of retail bottled water.

If you are limited to bottled water, try to purchase water that comes in glass bottles as the plastic bottles may contribute to your exposure of chemicals like BPA and phthalates. There are often delivery services that will drop off water at your home as well.

To get more water into your body, I suggest setting a quart jar of purified water next to your bed when you go to sleep at night. Then, before you even get out of bed in the morning, drink the whole quart. Watch what this simple morning ritual does to regulate your bowel movements and boost your energy. It will likely surprise and amaze you!

HERBAL TEAS

Many of us spend our time running around like crazy trying to accomplish more things in one day than is humanly possible. In order to complete the vast number of items on our lists, we often rely on pick-me-up beverages like coffee, black tea, and energy drinks. While some people seem to do fine with this "liquid cortisol" in their lives, others rely on it just to function, e.g., "I can't go anywhere until I've had my coffee!"

Some people can manage the effects of caffeine just fine, but for others, the constant consumption of caffeine will tax their livers. This may decrease the detoxification of toxic chemicals and weaken the system over time. Caffeine is also a diuretic, so it makes you pee out essential minerals. It also overstimulates your brain. Some people don't even realize how anxious and sleep deprived they are until they eliminate caffeine from their diet for a few weeks.

The studies on coffee are mixed: Some show that coffee can be beneficial, while others show that it can be harmful. It appears that the response is completely unique to the person. All I ask is that you remove all caffeine during the program to see how you feel. If your digestion, mood, focus, and sleep are much improved, leave it out. If you don't notice a difference, feel free to add your cup of brew back into your daily routine after the Elimination Diet program.

MANAGING CAFFEINE WITHDRAWAL

If you have terrible withdrawal headaches, you can add a cup of organic green tea to take the edge off. Just use the tea bag over again if you need a second cup. That will give you a bigger boost of the antioxidants, but far less of the caffeine.

It's important to stop and wonder how it is that we ended up with coffee as our crutch. There are indigenous cultures around the world that drink beverages made from mushrooms, bark, roots, shoots, leaves, and flowers that have energy-boosting, immune-supporting, and overall health-promoting effects. They have names like reishi mushroom, ashwagandha, astragalus, rhodiola, dandelion, burdock, licorice root, nettles, chamomile, and passion flower. Unlike caffeine, these seem to have a settling effect on the nervous system while boosting energy and cellular functions.

Sound too good to be true? It's not. Any ancient or recent text on herbal medicine will discuss the benefits of "adaptogenic" herbs. Adaptogenic plants produce and contain certain chemicals that can stabilize function and decrease cellular stress. Choosing these will help to promote calm and provide a stress-free source of energy.

If you haven't tried to make your own herbal teas yet, I highly recommend you start. It can be an incredibly tasty way to restore your health. Seek out a local herbalist and start asking questions—have fun by exploring and experimenting with new blends.

You can also look for herbal tea blends on the shelves of your local grocery store; just be sure they're organic and free of any flavorings. Detox blends and sleepy-time blends will help you relax and clear out harmful substances from your body. See a full list of herbal tea options in the Yes Foods: Foods to Eat list beginning on page 135.

FRESH COCONUT WATER

With more than 15 times the potassium of Gatorade and only half the sodium, coconut water is being touted as the best sports drink on the market. It's proven to be a superior source of hydration after workouts and competing in athletic events. Even when you're not hydrating post-workout, coconut water can have great benefits (plus, it tastes great!). Many people feel better after drinking coconut water and find that it gives them more energy and clearer thinking compared to regular drinking water.

The challenge is finding good-tasting coconut water that is in a nontoxic container and is free of any additives. There are many asceptic-packed (Tetra Paks) coconut waters and many canned options as well. Keep an eye on the cans, as they may have linings that contain endocrine disrupting chemicals like BPA.

Buying whole coconuts is a much better option if the coconuts are young and still have the husk attached. The young coconuts found wrapped in plastic are often nonorganic and usually have fungicide residues on them, which is why I don't recommend touching them with your bare hands. You can find whole green coconuts from Florida in some stores and they definitely can be purchased online, but the shipping costs can be quite high.

After years of searching, I have found two brands of bottled coconut water that meet most of my criteria. The best tasting and freshest 100 percent raw and organic coconut water in a bottle comes from the Harmless Harvest Company. Their product is not entirely perfect as they come in plastic bottles. If you are trying to reduce your plastic consumption, try Taste Nirvana coconut water, which you can find in glass bottles.

Now that you've been introduced to some of the featured ingredients during your detoxification days, let's explore what else you'll be eating and not eating in the first phase of the Elimination Diet.

FOODS TO EAT AND ELIMINATE DURING PHASE 1: DETOX

What you exclude during the Elimination Diet is just as important as what you include. If you don't exclude the irritants, you won't be successful with the program—it's that simple. Remember that you are the one who will benefit most if you can commit 100 percent to the diet. Don't deprive yourself of the gift of restored health.

You will use these lists during the first two phases of the Elimination Diet. In the third phase, you'll add the possible irritants back in slowly to test your reaction—I'll show you how it's done in chapter 9. In the Resources section, you'll find easy-to-copy versions of all the food lists. You can visit our website—WholeLifeNutrition.net—to download free PDFs of these food lists. I recommend placing them on your refrigerator for easy reference.

No Foods: Foods to Eliminate

ALL GRAINS:
Amaranth
Barley
Bread
Corn (see Corn list on page 134 for all types)
Millet
Oats/Oatmeal
Pasta
Quinoa
Rice
Rye
Sorghum

Spelt
Teff
Wheat

ALL LEGUMES:
Bean flours
Beans
Lentils
Peanuts
Peas

ALL DAIRY:
Butter and ghee
Cheese

Cottage cheese

Cream

Cream cheese

Evaporated milk

Ice cream

Milk

Sour cream

Sweetened condensed milk

Whey

Whipped cream

Yogurt

EGGS:

Chicken eggs

Duck eggs

Liquid eggs

Meringue

MEAT AND FISH:

All (except homemade Chicken
Stock, page 295)

ALL SOY:

Soy lecithin

Soy milk

Soy oil

Soy protein isolate

Soy protein powder

Tamari and soy sauce

Tempeh

Textured vegetable protein

Tofu

Vitamin E

CORN:

Baking powder

Corn flour

Corn on the cob

Corn tortillas

Cornmeal

Cornstarch

Dextrose

Food starch

Frozen corn

Grits

High-fructose corn syrup

Hominy

Maltodextrin

Masa

Polenta

Sorbitol

Vegetable gum

Vegetable protein

Vegetable starch

Xanthan gum

YEAST:

Autolyzed yeast extract

Baker's yeast

Brewer's yeast

Nutritional yeast

Vinegars (all except for raw
apple cider and coconut
vinegars)

ALL NUTS AND SEEDS:

Almond milk

Almonds

Cashews

Hazelnuts

Nut butters

Pecans

Pine nuts

Pumpkin seeds

Sesame seeds

Sunflower seeds
Walnuts

ALL CITRUS:
Grapefruit
Lemonade
Lemons
Limes
Orange juice
Oranges
Satsumas
Tangerines

NIGHTSHADE
VEGETABLES:
Cayenne pepper
Chili powder
Chipotle chile powder
Curry powder
Eggplant
Goji berries
Hot sauce
Mexican seasoning
Peppers (sweet and hot)
Potatoes
Taco seasoning
Tomatillos
Tomatoes

SUGAR:
Agave nectar
Cane sugar
Coconut nectar
Coconut sugar
Pure maple syrup
Raw honey
Sucanat

OTHER FOODS:
Alcohol
Caffeine
Chocolate
Refined vegetable oils

Yes Foods: Foods to Eat

MEATS:
Homemade Chicken Stock
    (page 295)

*FRUITS (JUICED, OR
PURÉED IN SMOOTHIES
DURING PHASE 1):*
Apples
Apricots (fresh only)
Avocados
Bananas
Berries (blueberries, blackberries,
    raspberries)
Cherries
Figs (fresh only)
Grapes
Melons
Nectarines and peaches
Papayas
Pears
Pineapple
Plums
Pomegranates

*VEGETABLES (JUICED, OR
PURÉED IN SMOOTHIES OR
SOUPS):*
Beets
Bok choy
Broccoli

Cabbage

Carrots

Cauliflower

Celeriac

Celery

Chard

Cilantro (coriander)

Collard greens

Cucumber

Fennel

Garlic

Ginger

Jerusalem artichokes (sunchoke)

Kale

Lettuce (all varieties except
   iceberg)

Mizuna

Mushrooms

Mustard greens

Onions

Parsley

Parsnips

Pumpkin

Rutabaga

Spinach

String beans

Sweet potatoes

Turnips

Watercress

Winter squash (all varieties)

Yams

Zucchini

GIVE THIS A TRY: MIZUNA

Mizuna is a dark leafy green otherwise known as Japanese mustard. It's slightly spicy, much like arugula, and is also part of the cruciferous vegetable family. Use it in salads, stir-fries, or soups. We grow it in our garden every year—it's incredibly easy to grow and fun to munch on!

SEA VEGETABLES:

Arame

Dulse

Hijiki

Kombu

Nori

OILS:

Extra-virgin olive oil

Virgin coconut oil

HERBAL TEAS:

Astragalus

Burdock

Chamomile

Dandelion root

Licorice

Mint

Nettle

Rooibos

Rose

Slippery elm

Tulsi (holy basil)

HERBS AND SPICES:

Allspice

Anise

Basil

Bay leaves

Black pepper (only freshly
ground)

Cinnamon

Cloves

Coriander

Cumin

Dill

Ginger (ground)

Nutmeg

Oregano

Thyme

Turmeric (ground)

OTHER INGREDIENTS:

Fresh coconut meat

Fresh coconut water

Raw organic apple cider vinegar

Raw organic coconut vinegar

PHASE 1: DETOX MEAL PLANS

The following sample meal plans will give you an idea of how to eat during the short detox phase of the plan. You can move these foods around as much as you'd like. Do you feel like soup for breakfast? Swap your straw for a spoon and dig in. We always recommend that you follow your gut instincts and consume the Elimination Diet–friendly foods that you are most attracted to eating in the moment.

Day 1

Breakfast: 2 cups Pineapple Green Smoothie (page 194)

Lunch: 2 to 4 cups Creamy Green Detox Soup (page 206)

Snack: 2 cups Purple Vegetable Juice (page 191)

Dinner: 2 to 4 cups Creamy Green Detox Soup (page 206)

Day 2

Breakfast: 2 cups Carrot-Cucumber-Ginger Juice (page 190)

Lunch: 2 to 4 cups Creamy Broccoli-Mushroom Soup (page 208)

Snack: 2 cups Red Cabbage and Berry Smoothie (page 193)

Dinner: 2 to 4 cups Creamy Cauliflower-Parsnip Soup (page 209)

PHASE 1 RECIPES

You'll have plenty of other recipes to choose from as you plan your meals during phase 1. Here's a complete list of recipes you can enjoy during this phase (see chapter 11 for recipes):

Carrot-Cucumber-Ginger Juice
Green Cleansing Juice
Purple Vegetable Juice
Beet-Fennel Juice
Very Berry Chia Smoothie
Red Cabbage and Berry Smoothie
Strawberry-Kale-Mint Smoothie
Pineapple Green Smoothie
Creamy Green Detox Soup
Carrot-Ginger-Shiitake Soup
Beet-Rosemary Detox Soup
Creamy Broccoli-Mushroom Soup
Creamy Cauliflower-Parsnip Soup
Baked Winter Squash
Cucumber-Mint Water
Warming Spice Tea
Nighttime Tea
Adrenal Support Tea
Chicken Stock
Vegetable-Seaweed Stock

FIVE STRATEGIES FOR A SUCCESSFUL DETOX

After guiding thousands of people on the Elimination Diet, I've been able to identify the most salient strategies for success. You can begin day one of your detox whenever you're ready, but as they say, "success leaves clues"—and I've got five important ones to share with you.

1. **Break out your journal.** During these first days of the plan, it's important to get into the habit of documenting how foods make you feel. This will grow even more important as we begin to test foods during the Reintroduction phase, but I want you to start practicing the act of listening to your body as soon as possible. Do you feel tired or energized? Are you having better bowel movements? Can you think clearly or do you feel a bit of cloudiness? Write it all down, and revisit your notes so you can monitor your progress.

2. **Don't focus on weight loss (even though it will happen).** The Elimination Diet is about eliminating your symptoms and consuming the most nourishing meals possible. When letting go of irritating foods and habits, many people will lose weight. Some lose between 5 and 7 pounds in the first week alone, and after twenty-eight days, the average weight loss is 15 to 16 pounds. Some people may need longer time or specific interventions to assist with weight loss. For example, you might need extra detox support—such as a specific supplement protocol—while others will need to reduce stress. Each individual will respond differently. The key point is to relax and enjoy your Elimination Diet adventure. Trust that your body will find balance when you determine the foods that create the best health for your unique system. Instead of thinking about all the weight you can lose, think about all of your suffering falling away as your energy and vitality increase.

3. **Pay attention to your bowels.** Every single moment of every single day, your bowels are talking. If they are quiet and calm, they are telling you that your diet is on the right track. If your bowels are gassy, crampy, or loose, there is a message for you there. Take mental notes or document specifics on your bowel movements (BMs) in your journal if you want to be a thorough diet detective.

4. **Learn to identify real hunger.** So many people eat to satisfy something other than hunger. They eat out of habit, to fulfill an emotional void, or to satisfy a biochemical craving for something like cheese, chocolate, or sugar. Before you give in to these temporary or false cravings, I want you to ask yourself: "Is this something I need right now to repair and replenish my body, or is there something else driving this feeling?" During the beginning days of the Elimination

Diet, you may have some incredibly strong desires to eat foods that really do not make sense to you. This is typical and should be expected. Instead of trying to overcome these desires, just satisfy them with healthful, satisfying foods that fall on your "Yes" list.

5. **Clear your calendar.** Holidays, birthdays, vacations, and office parties can be difficult to "survive" when you are on the Elimination Diet. If you can schedule the plan to fall over a period of time that is free from these events, you will increase your success rate exponentially. If you can't get around one of these events, be sure to bring some extra food to the event that you can eat.

8

PHASE 2:

Elimination—Days 3 to 14

After finishing phase 1 of the program, you should be on your way to feeling like a whole new person! Symptoms that have plagued you for years are starting to subside, and you are experiencing firsthand the incredible power of this program to change lives.

In Phase 2: Elimination, you will follow a baseline diet consisting of anti-inflammatory foods that normally don't cause an immune response in most people. If you've been experiencing joint and muscle pain, irritated bowels, headaches, skin outbreaks, foggy thinking, low energy, weight gain, insomnia, and depression, it's safe to say that inflammation is at play. To create healing and restore balance, we have to remove the inflammatory irritants and increase the beneficial nutrients coming into your body—we will achieve both during this phase.

For the next twelve days, I want you to focus on filling your plate with whole, organic, fresh foods. Hopefully, your home is already stocked with nourishing ingredients that will be transformed into beautiful, healing meals (see page 118 for a shopping list). Remember: You are eating to eliminate your symptoms while adding healthy foods to your diet.

During this phase, you can expect to feel a whole host of symptom changes, but how quickly you feel relief will depend on your symptoms and your unique system. Some people who follow the Elimination Diet feel worse on days 3 and 4. Others start to have the fog lift and their energy return by then. If you are suffering from migraines or asthma, look to days 5 to 7 as your turning point. Many people will have sinuses start to drain by

141

day 7, and joint pain should lighten up shortly after that if it hasn't already. Be patient; you will feel better if you are following the program.

The most important guide during this phase will be the food lists, which you'll find starting on page 154. What the lists don't tell you, however, is how to ensure you get the best quality foods. Throughout this chapter, I'll share strategies for selecting the most healing and healthful foods.

REMEMBER: THE TOP TRIGGERS STAY OUT

Congratulations—you've already made it through the first phase without some of the most irritating foods. You'll want to continue eliminating gluten, dairy, eggs, soy, corn, caffeine, and other potentially reactive foods. See the full list of foods to avoid during this phase starting on page 154.

PICK BETTER PROTEINS

Proteins, and the amino acids they are made of, are essential for countless reactions in the human body. Amino acids from foods such as meats, fish, nuts, and legumes are needed to make the digestive enzymes we use to access nutrients and the detoxification enzymes our body uses to process toxins. They are also used to make neurotransmitters like serotonin, melatonin, and dopamine that allow us to be happy, well rested, and calm. They play an essential role, too, with our intestinal cells, which die off every three days and need to be replaced by new cells. And where do the building blocks come from for all those new cells? Amino acids. In the simplest terms, if we do not have an adequate protein intake, our entire body cannot function properly.

In my practice, I've found that one of the most effective supplements I can recommend to people who have been in a state of disease for a while is amino acids. Just a few days of a broad-spectrum amino acid supplement and people feel better than they have after weeks of other supplements (see amino acids in the Resource section on page 305). I have seen this as an indication that people with chronic illnesses are often low on amino acids and do well with a little more protein.

The challenge with getting enough protein comes in finding good quality sources. Nuts, seeds, and beans are rich sources of proteins, but these are not always easy to digest (unless prepared properly) or easily tolerated. If you are someone who has digestive problems and suffers from gas, bloating, nausea, diarrhea, or constipation, you may want to consider emphasizing animal-based proteins over plant-based proteins during the Elimination Diet. You can first test your digestive function with the betaine HCL challenge (see Test Your Stomach Acid on page 33) and consider digestive enzymes. However, if your problems persist, I recommend getting your protein primarily from animal sources until your symptoms calm down.

Organic pasture-finished poultry (chicken and turkey) and wild fish (especially wild Alaskan salmon) have been shown to be great protein sources that are well tolerated by the majority of people doing the Elimination Diet. Let's look at how to get the best sources of poultry and fish.

Poultry

Choosing organic and/or pastured birds is of paramount importance. Poultry that is fed conventional feed will be consuming pesticides, which will end up in the meat and on the land, and eventually in your body if you eat it. Conventional birds are also often treated with antibiotics and antiparasitic medications that can contain toxic chemicals. Some nonorganic chicken producers may even inject tartrazine ("Yellow Dye Number 5") and salt mixtures into the packaged meat to give it better color and texture.

Until 2010, it was common practice for many large chicken producers to treat their chickens with a parasite medication containing arsenic. This led to arsenic levels in chicken that would be considered unsafe for long-term consumption. As of this writing, there is a voluntary moratorium on some of the more dangerous arsenic medications, but certain producers are still using toxic medications. Avoid these by selecting organically produced poultry.

Fish

There are many things to consider when choosing what fish to eat. What type of fish it is, where it was caught, and how it was caught will affect the quality of the fish, the amount of chemicals in it, and the global sustainability of those fish stocks for future generations.

Because environmental conditions and fish populations change each year, I recommend familiarizing yourself with the Seafood Watch program, a fantastic resource offered through the Monterey Bay Aquarium. On their website (seafoodwatch.org), you can find the most up-to-date information on the safest and smartest fish to buy. They even have downloadable pocket guides to assist you with your choices.

Look to their Super Green List for fish selections that will be good for your health and good for the oceans. Fish on this list will have lower mercury levels, provide at least 250 milligrams of omega-3s, and be classified as sustainable. In the past, Atlantic mackerel, Pacific sardines, and Alaskan salmon have made the cut—but check the website for the most current information.

When purchasing fish, make sure it is firm and does not smell too fishy. Smelly or soft fish can indicate high amine levels that may contribute to food reactions.

GET GOOD GRAINS

With gluten gone, does that mean all grains are out? No. During this phase, you can get good-quality carbohydrates from brown rice, wild rice, and quinoa (preferably organic and sprouted).

People with blood sugar issues like type 1 diabetes and severe insulin resistance, and/or starch digestion problems may do better with a grain-free or low-grain diet. Others will often feel better when they include some grains in their diet.

There is a lot of chatter on the web and in books regarding grain-free diets as the solution to our rising rates of diabetes, obesity, and autoimmune diseases. If I had not seen numerous clients lower their blood sugar levels, body weight, cholesterol, and improve their autoimmune conditions and irritated bowel problems while still eating grains, I might believe them. When grains are eaten in moderation and in balance with other nourishing foods, they can be perfectly healthy. They're even better for you when you soak, sprout, or ferment them. Try our dosa recipe on page 222 and see what you think.

The trick with grains is that they must be gluten-free during the Elimination Diet process, which can be a difficult thing to guarantee. Over the years, I have seen people have gluten-identical reactions to millet, sorghum, oats, and buckwheat. At first I thought it may have been that these people had separate reactions to these grains. But as my clients report more cross-contamination cases to me and the literature starts revealing more case studies, I believe that cross contamination of gluten is behind most cases of these reactions.

Most people will do well on the grains listed in this program. If you continue to have symptoms of gas, nausea, bloating, and erratic bowel movements, you may want to try going bean-free first, and then grain- and bean-free. Once the gut is healed and the beneficial bacteria restored, most people can digest and enjoy gluten-free whole grains and beans in their diets.

EXPANDING YOUR VEGETABLE REPERTOIRE

You already learned a bit about the incredible phytochemicals found in vegetables (see page 128), but now I want to call your attention to the palate-pleasing potential they hold. It's time think beyond iceberg lettuce and canned cream corn. No more fast-food salads that lack the nutrients you need for your detoxification and elimination experience. Here are some tips for exploring and enjoying vegetables this phase:

- **Get to know some new greens.** Have you tried arugula or mustard greens? They're peppery and bright in flavor, and also stimulate the liver to produce detoxification enzymes! Or try romaine, red romaine, mizuna, red- or green-leaf, and butter-leaf lettuces to liven up your salads.
- **Try this snack on for size.** Instead of letting opened packages of chips, cookies, and crackers gather on your household countertop, try fresh veggies instead. Slice cucumbers, radishes, kohlrabi, carrots, and celery and place them in jars of water in your refrigerator. They'll be waiting for you, fresh and crispy.
- **Swap good for great.** Spinach and chard are excellent greens, but they're higher in oxalates, which can contribute to joint pain, irritability, and intestinal upset in some people if eaten often. During the Elimination Diet, opt for collards and black kale in soups, salads, and smoothies.

- **Eat these green giants.** Green beans and broccoli will provide folates, vitamin K, magnesium, amino acids, and more phytochemicals than you can shake a stick at.
- **Enjoy digestion-friendly starches.** Kabocha and spaghetti squashes will provide some healthy, easily digested starches that can help to satisfy cravings for unhealthy carbs and quell your hunger at the same time.
- **Dig these natural sweeteners.** As long as you do not have bloating and bowel problems, butternut squash and yams will be great tools for creating sweet and satisfying snacks, side dishes, desserts, and even main courses.

If there is one thing you can do to improve your health, it is to eat more vegetables. Eating an average of eight servings a day of fruits and vegetables can lower your risk for heart attack or stroke by 30 percent.

Don't be afraid to expand your vegetable horizon during this phase. You might discover something new in the recipes or on the list of approved foods—give it a try!

EAT OPTIMAL FATS

Fats are used in every cell of the body, where they help form part of the cells' walls. They're also used as fuel for energy, help us make many of our hormones, and form our brain tissue. You need healthy fats to maintain a healthy body.

Unfortunately, many people are getting their daily fats from refined oils that are extracted with the use of solvents like hexane in their production process. Once extracted, these oils are heavily used in processed foods. The most common are canola, cottonseed, soy, and corn oils. Around 90 percent of the crops used to produce these oils are genetically modified to sustain the spraying of large amounts of herbicides.

When you consume foods containing canola, cottonseed, soy, and corn oils, or use them to cook, you are likely ingesting both the herbicides and solvents. These substances can go on to alter your gut flora and irritate your intestines. If that isn't bad enough, many of the polyunsaturated oils like canola, safflower, flax, and corn oil will easily spoil in storage or while you are cooking with them.

HOW FAST DOES OIL SPOIL?

If you've ever tried fresh-pressed oil, you know it tastes almost nothing like what you can buy on store shelves. I used to have a group of friends who worked at a flax oil company, and I was lucky enough to get invited over to try some of their fresh-pressed oil. They poured some of the oil in a sample cup and I took a sip and was blown away. The taste was amazing: nutty and light with an almost sweet aftertaste. As we were talking, I would periodically take another sip of the oil. In less than 5 minutes, I began to notice a change in the flavor. The sweetness had been replaced with a bitter aftertaste. About 20 minutes later, the bitterness had turned to an almost metallic taste. The contrast was unmistakable. The bottom line: Oil can spoil, and when it does, its nutritional properties begin to change. To prevent oil from spoiling:

- Store it away from light, in a dark cupboard or pantry. Also look to buy oils in tinted glass to minimize light exposure. If you have flax oil, it must be stored in the refrigerator with the cap on tight.
- Select a storage space away from the stove and oven, if possible. Heat can accelerate spoilage.
- If it has turned, toss it. Consuming rancid oil can increase inflammation.

To avoid rancid oils and excessive chemical exposure, during this phase, you will remove all oils, except extra-virgin cold-pressed organic olive and coconut oils. Here's why they make the cut:

Olive oil is a monounsaturated fat that has very protective antioxidant compounds that keep it from spoiling as quickly as other monounsaturated fats. Some of these protective phenolic compounds (protocatechuic acid and oleuropein) have been shown to reduce the incidence of heart disease and type 2 diabetes.

Coconut oil contains saturated fats (like lauric acid) that are stable at higher heats and don't spoil easily. Lauric acid is a medium-chain triglyceride or MCT, which doesn't demand much from your digestive system. Because coconut oil contains MCTs, it can be quickly absorbed into the body and burned as fuel more easily than other fats. Athletes in my practice will commonly add MCTs to their smoothies for an extra boost of healthy fats that will give them sustained energy without adding weight to their waistlines. MCTs found in coconut oil also kill of harmful yeasts in the GI tract, which will help balance the microbiome.

SWITCH OUT YOUR SWEETENERS

All sweeteners are on the "no" list, except coconut sugar and coconut nectar, maple syrup, raw honey, stevia, and dates (and they must be whole dates, not date pieces).

Like most people, you probably enjoy sweet-tasting foods on occasion, maybe even on more occasions than you'd like to admit. The problem with most candies, cookies, and baked goods is that they're full of refined sweeteners. Refined sweeteners, like white sugar and high-fructose corn syrup, have been heavily processed into a form that is lacking in nutrients and fiber, but full of quick-absorbing carbs. This is a recipe for inflammation. When you eat refined sugars, you will experience extreme spikes in blood sugar and increased inflammation, and you'll have wiped out opportunities to eat more nutrient-dense foods.

Consuming foods full of the standard-use white sugar also increases your exposure to GM crops. Unless a sugar says "100 percent cane sugar," you can be assured that more than 90 percent of the sugar is coming from GM sugar beet crops and is contaminated with glyphosate and other chemicals.

The good news is you don't have to give up the treat of sweetness; you just need to realize that there are healthier options provided by nature. These are the sweet saps of maple and palm trees; nectar from flowers; sweet leaves; and the fruits of tropical palm trees.

Keep in mind that even though these sweeteners are natural, this does not mean you should indulge in them freely. If you've been eating a diet with plenty of refined carbohydrates and refined sugars, your sense of how much sugar you really need to satisfy a sweet tooth is likely warped. When you give your body and your taste buds a break from processed sugars, you will be amazed at how incredible the natural flavors in fresh fruits and vegetables begin to taste.

Use these approved sweeteners with care, but also consider keeping them out of your diet through the end of phase 2; do this and you will allow yourself to become truly reconnected with your desire for sweetness.

Coconut Sugar and Coconut Nectar

The sap of coconut trees can be sustainably harvested and used either as a liquid product (coconut nectar) or a dried powder (coconut sugar). Coconut sugar is less likely to spike blood sugar because it is high in specific long-chain sugars called fructooligosaccharides (FOS), and a soluble fiber called inulin, which give it a lower glycemic index. FOS and inulin are commonly used as food (prebiotics) by bacteria in our intestinal tracts. If you have lots of gas and bloating due to a bacterial overgrowth in your intestines, you may want to limit coconut sugar consumption to small amounts.

Maple Syrup

Before the introduction of sugar in North America, residents of the United States relied on the sap of maple trees to satisfy their sweet cravings. Like coconut nectar, maple syrup is one of the least-refined sweeteners available. It also contains the minerals zinc, potassium, manganese, and calcium. I recommend the darker grade B maple syrup for its richer taste and mineral content.

Raw Honey

As bees travel from flower to flower gathering nectar and pollen, they will concentrate other chemicals found in those plants as well. When you choose raw honey, you will get more pinostrobin, a potent compound that ramps up your cells' detoxification and antioxidant functions (it's almost as powerful as the miraculous sulforaphane from broccoli sprouts).

Most people will tolerate small amounts of honey, but those with IBS and SIBO could find it bothersome. Certain varieties of honey are less troublesome than others. While alfalfa, raspberry, and clover honeys are recommended by SIBO experts, I recommend using wild clover honey, as it is likely to contain less pesticide residues. Just pay attention to your journal entries when it comes to honey and any other foods. If you continue to notice digestive distress after eating honey, you may want to limit your intake.

Stevia

Stevia is an herb that is an excellent, natural replacement for sugar. We grow this amazing plant in our garden. If you ever get a chance to taste a raw stevia leaf, you will know exactly why it is used as a sweetener—it is more than 100 times sweeter than sugar.

The great thing about stevia is it can provide a satisfying sweet flavor without spiking blood sugar. And, unlike sugar, stevia may protect your teeth from cavities. The tricky part in using stevia is it is extremely difficult to use as a sugar replacement in recipes because it is so sweet. Just be forewarned if you're considering using it in baking. There are literally entire cookbooks to educate you on using stevia in baking.

If you've never tried stevia, start with just a few bites of any foods containing this sweetener; it has an interesting aftertaste, which some love and others don't.

Dates

Poor dates. For the longest time they have gotten a bad reputation. Due to some poorly done research, people have assumed dates have an extremely high glycemic index and spike blood sugar in an extreme way. Thankfully, recent science is showing this is not so much the case.

As a whole food, they contain fiber, magnesium, manganese, and even a small amount of protein. Dates should not be eaten in large amounts, but a little goes a long way. They're great in desserts, smoothies, or just eaten raw.

It's important to remember to not purchase date pieces, but only whole dates. Date pieces are often sprinkled with flour that can be contaminated with gluten.

Dates contain oligosaccharides that may cause trouble for people with SIBO and IBS.

THE SPICE IS RIGHT

Spices can add incredible and essential flavors to food. And if you know the right kind to buy, you can add flavor without triggering any type of food reaction. Here's what to shop for:

Individual herbs and spices, not mixes: If you buy herb and spice mixes, you risk anticaking agents being used in the product. Anticaking agents are used to prevent individual spices from clumping together, and the most commonly used one is wheat flour.

Buy whole individual herbs and spices instead and make your own mixes. We have mortar and pestles and graters in our kitchen at all times to process our herbs and spices. Not only does it ensure that we're not getting exposed to unnecessary ingredients, but the flavor of freshly ground cinnamon, nutmeg, or ginger is out of this world.

Spices made without additives and preservatives: Other additives and preservatives may be added to make sure that volatile oils found in herbs and spices do not spoil. While this is good for the product, it is not always good for your body: Some preservatives and additives can cause irritation and lead to a food reaction. Check the label.

Organic varieties: It is imperative to choose organic herbs and spices over conventional products. According to an article from the Organic Consumers Association, "Virtually all conventional spices sold in the United States are fumigated [sterilized] with hazardous chemicals that are banned in Europe."

Many spices sourced from around the globe will come from places that have less stringent regulations on harmful chemicals like pesticides and heavy metals. Buying organic will lower your exposure to chemicals tremendously.

Of course, the best option of all is to grow your own fresh herbs. The best starter herbs include mint and oregano. They are so easy to grow that you have to plant them in places where you don't mind if they spread—a ceramic pot on your front porch is one of the best ways to grow them.

VINEGAR

There's a reason why vinegar has been around for more than 10,000 years—it's one of the most versatile liquids ever discovered. It's been used as a preservative, a solvent, a pickling agent, and more. And of course, it's the other half of the most commonly used dressing in many cultures: oil and vinegar.

Hippocrates once touted vinegar's medicinal qualities, which derive partly from its acidic properties. The acidity of vinegar can assist your own stomach acid in the breakdown of proteins, help release nutrients from foods, and stimulate the release of digestive enzymes.

THE POWER COUPLE: OIL AND VINEGAR

Native cultures were quite wise in using acidic vinegar on their salad greens, many of which were and still are tough to digest. Marinating salad greens in an acid helps to break apart some of their cell walls, releasing nutritious plant chemicals and making them more available for absorption into our bodies. Many of these plant chemicals cannot be absorbed without other fats in the diet as well. Enter olive oil. The addition of this versatile and tasty oil (full of good fat) helps unlock the best possible nutrition from your salad.

During the Elimination Diet, you will be excluding the use of all vinegars except for raw apple cider vinegar and raw coconut vinegar. It's important to stick to using only these two vinegars since there are multiple aspects of other vinegars that could cause a reaction. You could react to an additive or preservative, the food from which the vinegar is fermented, or the organism that is used to ferment the vinegar. Here are some common examples of vinegars that my clients have reacted to and why:

- Malt vinegars, which can be fermented from gluten grains and have gluten in them
- Balsamic vinegars, likely due to higher concentrations of phenylethylamines and sulfites
- Plum vinegar, because of its high-fructose corn syrup
- Rice vinegar, due to its sugar content

While people with Crohn's disease, migraines, anxiety, hyperactivity, and/or a known amine sensitivity may want to avoid all vinegars, the two vinegars I have found to be the most tolerated by the general population are coconut and raw apple cider vinegar. Both are derived from hypoallergenic foods and are fermented by an organism known as "the mother" that appears to be better tolerated by most people.

WHAT TO DRINK

During the diet, you will remove all beverages except purified water, decaffeinated green tea and herbal teas (with no additives or flavorings), and fresh vegetable juices. This means no coffee, black tea, energy drinks, sports drinks, soda, or alcohol.

We remove coffee and caffeinated teas because they contain chemicals that can slow down your ability to detoxify, and are a common cause of irritability and insomnia (more on this on page 64). Most people will also feel compelled to add certain items to coffees and teas that are excluded during the Elimination Diet. These include cream, sugar, milk, nondairy creamers, and flavored sweeteners.

Sodas, sport drinks, and other processed beverages often contain sweeteners, additives, preservatives, and coloring that can contribute to symptoms including rashes, irritable bowel disease, anxiety, hyperactivity, headaches, and more. Combining a bit of organic pineapple with coconut water and a dash of sea salt in a blender can provide a healthier alternative to sports drinks.

Many alcoholic beverages have ingredients that may contain gluten, artificial flavors and/or colors, or preservatives. Some examples:

- Wine: sulfites and amines
- Beer: gluten from barley
- Scotch and rye whiskey: gluten from wheat and rye
- Gin and vodka: gluten from barley or rye; also can contain corn
- Alcoholic mixes: high-fructose corn syrup, artificial colors

While sweetened, caffeinated, and alcoholic beverages will dehydrate your body and increase the excretion of essential minerals into your urine, purified water and coconut water do the exact opposite. They allow you to stay hydrated all day long. Staying properly hydrated during the Elimination Diet is imperative, as it will help your body flush toxins out from your kidneys and in your sweat. Drinking replenishing beverages will also ensure that you have plenty of blood flow to transport nutrients, remove toxins from your brain, and transport oxygen to every tissue in your body. The intestinal tract stays pliable and is less prone to damage when we are well hydrated as well.

Herbal teas and vegetable juices will add essential phytochemicals to boost your immune system, support each and every cell to process toxins and produce antioxidants, and keep your energy level high.

FOODS TO EAT AND AVOID DURING PHASE 2: ELIMINATION

Below are the foods to avoid and include during phase 2. Visit our website, WholeLifeNutrition.net, for simple, printable phase lists. We suggest printing out this list and posting it to your refrigerator.

No Foods: Foods to Eliminate

GLUTEN:
Buckwheat (cross contaminated with gluten)
Kamut
Lentils (cross contaminated with gluten)
Millet (cross contaminated with gluten)
Oats (cross contaminated with gluten)
Rye
Sorghum (cross contaminated with gluten)
Spelt
Triticale
Wheat

DAIRY:
Butter and ghee
Cheese
Cottage cheese
Cream
Cream cheese
Evaporated milk
Ice cream
Milk
Sour cream
Sweetened condensed milk
Whey
Whipped cream
Yogurt

EGGS:
Chicken eggs
Duck eggs
Liquid eggs
Meringue

MEAT:
Beef
Lard
Pork
Tallow

SOY:
Soy lecithin
Soy milk
Soy oil
Soy protein isolate

Soy protein powder
Tamari and soy sauce
Tempeh
Textured vegetable protein
Tofu
Vitamin E (with soy oil)

CORN:
Baking powder
Corn flour
Corn on the cob
Corn tortillas
Cornmeal
Cornstarch
Dextrose
Food starch
Frozen corn
Grits
High-fructose corn syrup
Hominy
Maltodextrin
Masa
Polenta
Sorbitol
Vegetable gum
Vegetable protein
Vegetable starch
Xanthan gum

YEAST:
Autolyzed yeast extract
Baker's yeast
Brewer's yeast
Nutritional yeast
Vinegars (all except for raw
    apple cider and coconut
    vinegars)

NUTS:
Almond butter
Almonds
Brazil nuts
Cashew butter
Cashews
Hazelnuts
Macadamia nuts
Peanut butter (actually legumes)
Peanuts (actually legumes)
Pecans
Pistachios
Walnuts

CITRUS:
Grapefruit
Lemonade
Lemons
Limes
Orange juice
Oranges
Satsumas
Tangerines

NIGHTSHADE VEGETABLES:
Cayenne pepper
Chili powder
Chipotle chile powder
Curry powder
Eggplant
Hot sauce
Mexican seasoning
Peppers (sweet and hot)
Potatoes
Taco seasoning
Tomatillos
Tomatoes

SUGAR:

Agave nectar

Beet sugar

Cane sugar

Sucanat

OTHER FOODS:

Alcohol

Caffeine

Chocolate

Refined vegetable oil

Sesame

Yes Foods: Foods to Eat

WHOLE GRAINS:

Brown rice

Brown rice flour

Quinoa

Quinoa flour

White jasmine rice

Wild rice

LEGUMES:

Adzuki beans

Black beans

Garbanzo bean flour
(preferably organic and
sprouted)

Garbanzo beans

Lima beans

Mung beans

Pinto and pink beans

White beans

MEATS AND FISH:

Anchovies

Black cod

Chicken (organic)

Duck

Goose

Herring

Lamb (organic)

Pheasant

Pollock

Turkey (organic)

Venison

Wild salmon

Wild scallops

FRUITS:

Apples

Apricots (fresh or dried with no
added preservatives)

Bananas

Berries (blueberries, blackberries,
raspberries)

Cherries

Dates (fresh or dried with no
preservatives or additives)

Figs (fresh and dried with no
preservatives or additives)

Grapes

Melons

Nectarines and peaches

Papayas

Pears

Pineapple

Plums

Pomegranates

VEGETABLES:

Artichoke

Asparagus

Avocados
Beets
Bok choy
Broccoli
Brussels sprouts
Cabbage
Carrots
Cauliflower
Celeriac
Celery
Chard
Cilantro (coriander)
Collard greens
Cucumber
Fennel
Garlic
Ginger
Jerusalem artichokes (sunchokes)
Kale
Lettuce (all varieties except
   iceberg)
Mizuna
Mushrooms
Mustard greens
Onions
Parsley
Parsnips
Peas (sugar snap, snow, frozen,
   and dried split)
Pickles (homemade without
   peppers)
Pumpkin
Rutabaga
Spinach
String beans

Sweet potatoes
Turnips
Watercress
Winter squash (all varieties)
Yams
Zucchini

SEA VEGETABLES:
Arame
Dulse
Hijiki
Kombu
Nori

SEEDS AND BUTTERS:
Raw chia seeds
Raw flaxseeds
Raw hemp seeds
Raw pine nuts
Raw pumpkin seed butter
Raw pumpkin seeds
Raw sunflower seeds

OILS:
Extra-virgin olive oil
Virgin coconut oil

SWEETENERS:
Coconut nectar
Coconut sugar
Pure maple syrup
Raw honey

HERBAL TEAS:
Astragalus
Burdock
Chamomile

Dandelion root

Licorice

Mint

Nettle

Rooibos

Rose

Slippery elm

Tulsi (holy basil)

HERBS AND SPICES:

Allspice

Anise

Basil

Bay leaves

Black pepper (only freshly
   ground)

Cinnamon

Cloves

Coriander

Cumin

Dill

Ginger (ground)

Nutmeg

Oregano

Thyme

Turmeric (ground)

OTHER INGREDIENTS:

Agar flakes and powder

Arrowroot powder (make sure
   it comes from a gluten-free
   facility)

Coconut aminos

Coconut milk (canned, organic)

Fresh coconut meat

Fresh coconut water

Kudzu

Raw organic apple cider vinegar

Raw organic coconut vinegar

Raw organic vanilla powder

PHASE 2: ELIMINATION MEAL PLANS AND RECIPE LIST

We've helped take the guesswork out of meal planning for you during this phase. Use these sample days to get you on track with how to eat and plan for your meals, though we strongly encourage you to listen to your own body. Some days you might not need as much food, at times you might have cravings for a meat-based meal, and at other times you might wish to eat only raw vegetables. The healthiest meal plans will be the ones you devise on a day-to-day basis from the allowable foods during each phase. Once you clear out the processed-food clutter from your diet, it will become easier and easier to listen to what your body really needs each and every day. Feel free to swap or move around meals as you'd like.

Day 3

Breakfast: 2 cups Simple Vegetable Soup (page 213)

Lunch: Summer Salad with Blueberry Vinaigrette (page 230), ½ cup cooked chicken or wild salmon

Snack: 1 to 2 cups Red Cabbage and Berry Smoothie (page 193)

Dinner: Black Bean, Yam, and Avocado Tacos (page 255)

Day 4

Breakfast: Chicken-Apple Breakfast Sausage (page 202) over lettuce leaves, topped with Fresh Broccoli Sprouts (page 301)

Lunch: 2 to 4 cups Creamy Green Detox Soup (page 206)

Snack: 1 to 2 cups Beet-Fennel Juice (page 191)

Dinner: Herb-Roasted Wild Salmon (page 257), Coconut-Cinnamon Roasted Sweet Potatoes (page 243), baby arugula salad with Green Goddess Dressing (page 273)

Day 5

Breakfast: Coconut-Quinoa Breakfast Porridge (page 198)

Lunch: 2 cups Simple Vegetable Soup (page 213)

Snack: 2 Chai-Spiced Sunflower Truffles (page 282)

Dinner: Spiced Chicken and Yams (page 266), baby arugula salad with Green Goddess Dressing (page 273)

Day 6

Breakfast: 2 to 4 cups Strawberry-Kale-Mint Smoothie (page 194)

Lunch: Mustard-Herb Lamb Burger (page 270) wrapped in a lettuce leaf with cucumber slices, fresh mint leaves, and a dollop of Coconut Sour Cream (page 277)

Snack: 2 Chai-Spiced Sunflower Truffles (page 282)

Dinner: Adzuki Bean and Rice Salad (page 248) served over lettuce leaves, Baked Winter Squash (page 243)

Day 7

Breakfast: Turkey, Kale, and Carrot Hash (page 199) with Baked Winter
Squash (page 243)

Lunch: Healing Cabbage and Chicken Soup (page 214)

Snack: apple slices dipped in pumpkin seed butter

Dinner: Spring Salad with Snap Peas, Salmon, and Radishes (page 230),
cooked quinoa

Day 8

Breakfast: Sweet Potato–Kale Hash (page 200), topped with toasted
pumpkin seeds

Lunch: Creamy Green Detox Soup (page 206) topped with cooked
salmon and Fresh Broccoli Sprouts (page 301)

Snack: Vanilla-Coconut Snowballs (page 281) and a handful of fresh or
frozen blueberries

Dinner: Chicken and Vegetable Stir-Fry (page 261), Vegetable and Rice
Nori Rolls (page 250)

Day 9

Breakfast: Spiced Seed Granola (page 204) with Vanilla Hemp Milk
(page 290) and sliced bananas and fresh blueberries

Lunch: Sweet Potato, Fennel, and Chicken Stew (page 218), ¼ cup
Pickled Cauliflower, Carrots, and Green Beans (page 297)

Snack: Strawberry-Kale-Mint Smoothie (page 194)

Dinner: Pomegranate Chicken Tacos (page 259)

Day 10

Breakfast: Creamy Rice Cereal (page 198) topped with fresh blueberries
and cinnamon

Lunch: Garlic Chicken Salad (page 236)

Snack: Salt and Pepper Kale Chips (page 244)

Dinner: Mustard-Herb Lamb Burger (page 270) wrapped in a lettuce leaf with cucumber slices, fresh mint leaves, and a dollop of Coconut Sour Cream (page 277)

Day 11

Breakfast: 2 to 3 cups Red Cabbage and Berry Smoothie (page 193)
Lunch: Sweet Potato, Fennel, and Chicken Stew (page 218), ¼ cup Pickled Cauliflower, Carrots, and Green Beans (page 297)
Snack: Salt and Pepper Kale Chips (page 244)
Dinner: quinoa pasta or zucchini noodles with Nightshade-Free Pasta Sauce (page 278) cooked with ground organic turkey, organic baby green salad

Day 12

Breakfast: Pineapple Green Smoothie (page 194)
Lunch: Lamb-Quinoa Breakfast Hash (page 201)
Snack: Pumpkin Seed Butter Energy Bar (page 282)
Dinner: Vegetable Chicken Bake (page 263), organic baby green salad with Zucchini-Dill Vinaigrette (page 276)

Day 13

Breakfast: Turkey, Kale, and Carrot Hash (page 199)
Lunch: Beet-Rosemary Detox Soup (page 208)
Snack: Pumpkin Seed Butter Energy Bar (page 282)
Dinner: Herb-Roasted Wild Salmon (page 257), Baked Winter Squash (page 243), organic baby green salad with Blueberry Vinaigrette (page 272)

Day 14

Breakfast: Coconut-Quinoa Breakfast Porridge (page 198)
Lunch: Spring Salad with Snap Peas, Salmon, and Radishes (page 230)

Snack: Salt and Pepper Kale Chips (page 244)
Dinner: Whole Roasted Chicken with Rosemary (page 265), Baked
   Winter Squash (page 243), Dill Pickled Turnips (page 298), steamed
   green beans

PHASE 2 RECIPES

When you get to chapter 11, you'll notice many other recipes that you'll be
able to enjoy during this phase. Here's the complete list:

Creamy Rice Cereal
Coconut-Quinoa Breakfast Porridge
Turkey, Kale, and Carrot Hash
Sweet Potato–Kale Hash
Lamb-Quinoa Breakfast Hash
Chicken-Apple Breakfast Sausages
Celeriac-Rutabaga Hash Browns
Spiced Seed Granola
Adzuki Bean and Sea Vegetable Soup
White Bean, Wild Rice, and Kale Soup
Simple Vegetable Soup
Healing Cabbage and Chicken Soup
Chicken Vegetable Soup
Turkey Vegetable Soup
Sweet Potato, Fennel, and Chicken Stew
Harvest Squash Soup
Quinoa and Black Bean Dosas
Brown Rice Tortillas
Banana Muffins
Spring Salad with Snap Peas, Salmon, and Radishes
Summer Salad with Blueberry Vinaigrette
Roasted Delicata Squash Salad with Apples and Toasted Pumpkin Seeds
Napa Cabbage Salad with Ginger-Cilantro Dressing
Crunchy Romaine Salad with Italian Herb Dressing
Garlic Chicken Salad
Cucumber-Mint Salad

Garlic-Braised Collard Greens
Sautéed Kale with Shiitake Mushrooms
Butternut Squash and Sage Stuffing
Cauliflower-Parsnip Mash with Fresh Herbs
Roasted Root Vegetables
Roasted Brussels Sprouts and Cauliflower
Coconut-Cinnamon Roasted Sweet Potatoes
Salt and Pepper Kale Chips
Basic Brown Rice
Basic Wild Rice
Basic Quinoa
Adzuki Bean and Rice Salad
Basil-Radish-Quinoa Salad
Vegetable and Rice Nori Rolls
Mung Bean and Rice Kitcheree
Moroccan-Spiced Vegetable Stew
Black Bean, Yam, and Avocado Tacos
Herb-Roasted Wild Salmon
Pomegranate Chicken Tacos
Chicken Fried Cauliflower "Rice"
Chicken and Vegetable Stir-Fry
Chicken-Spinach Burgers
Vegetable Chicken Bake
Whole Roasted Chicken with Rosemary
Spiced Chicken and Yams
Brined Turkey Breast
Turkey-Herb-Quinoa Meatballs
Mustard-Herb Lamb Burgers
Blueberry Vinaigrette
Green Goddess Dressing
Creamy Garlic–Hemp Seed Dressing
Creamy Sunflower Seed–Parsley Dressing
Ginger-Apple Dressing
Zucchini-Dill Vinaigrette
Coconut Sour Cream
Nightshade-Free Pasta Sauce

Fresh Berries with Whipped Vanilla Coconut Cream

Vanilla-Coconut Snowballs

Chai-Spiced Sunflower Truffles

Pumpkin Seed Butter Energy Bars

Peachy Coconut Creamsicles

Vanilla Hemp Milk

Pickled Cauliflower, Carrots, and Green Beans

Dill Pickled Turnips

Rainbow Kraut

Fresh Broccoli Sprouts

9

PHASE 3:

Reintroduction—Days 15 and On

You've made it to the Reintroduction phase—congratulations! If you're like most of my clients, the past couple of weeks have probably been transformational for you. Many of my clients tell me that they never knew they could feel so good. They had been living with chronic inflammation and uncomfortable symptoms for so many years that they believed that was normal for them. After two weeks of eating healing foods and avoiding reactive foods, I hope you're enjoying your new normal, too! Think of the great gifts you've given yourself by following this program: a calm, cool immune system and a replenished, balanced intestinal tract. You've lost weight, reduced inflammation, and have lessened or eliminated symptoms like bloating, bowel upset, joint pain, fatigue, and perhaps many others.

Now it's time for the truly exciting part of the Elimination Diet—over the next few weeks, you are going to create a customized diet for yourself. You will learn which foods work for your unique body chemistry, and which don't. During this phase, you will add foods back in, one by one, to see if you are having a reaction. Reintroduction includes two basic steps—first, you'll test a food, and then you'll document any reaction. From there, you'll move on to the next food. If this sounds complicated, don't worry; I'll walk you through the process step by step.

Before you begin phase 3, reintroducing potentially triggering foods, I want you to take an honest inventory of how you're feeling. Answering these questions will help create an even greater level of customization of the Elimination Diet (it will almost be as though you've come into my office for personalized treatment). Ask yourself these questions:

- Have my symptoms subsided?
- Do I have more energy?
- Has my mood improved?
- Have I lost weight?
- Do my hair and skin look better?

HELP—I'M STILL NOT FEELING BETTER!

If you have not experienced any symptom changes by day 15, it is time to pause and consider what might be behind your lack of success. Using the chart below, find your symptom and the steps you should take to help alleviate it. It's highly recommended that you follow the steps outlined here until you experience relief from your symptoms (follow them in the order listed). If you reintroduce foods before your system is calm, you won't know the true source of your reactions.

I am still experiencing: fatigue, joint pain, back pain, headaches, and/or foggy thinking.

Possible culprit: You could have missed a source of irritation or be lacking in key nutrients to decrease your symptoms.

Action steps:

1. **Check for cross contamination.** Hidden sources of irritant foods are the prime reason clients don't experience relief from these symptoms. Gluten, soy, and corn are likely to sneak into your diet unbeknownst to you. Visit our website, WholeLifeNutrition .net, to check out our Hidden Sources of Contamination page.

2. **Check for toxic exposures.** Here are three things to consider that may be contributing to your inflammation:
   - Nonorganic foods—especially meats.
   - Personal care items: lotions, creams, perfumes, cologne, hair products, and so on that have irritant chemicals in them. See Endocrine Disrupting Chemicals (EDCs) on page 75 for more details.
   - Household products: Dryer sheets, scented cleaning agents, pesticides, laundry and dishwashing detergent, off-gassing

from new building materials (paints, furniture, flooring, etc.). Apply your diet detective skills to your environment. If you recall Jimmy's story from chapter 4 (page 70), he felt better when he went camping. Has anything changed in your environment? Is there a time when you've felt relief from your symptoms?

3. **Look to the supplement section for additional nutrient support.** A lack of vitamin D, essential fatty acids, and magnesium can impair the healing process, while supplementing with Meriva can reduce inflammation (see Supplements to Support the Elimination Diet on page 107).

I am still experiencing: gas, nausea, bloating, diarrhea, constipation, and/or skin conditions.

Possible culprit: You may have an underlying deficiency in substances important to digestion, or an unknown intolerance to foods that aren't eliminated during the first two phases of the diet.

Action steps:

1. Test your gastric acid to see if you are deficient (see Test Your Stomach Acid on page 33). If you are deficient, take betaine HCL.
2. Try digestive enzyme supplementation (see page 112).
3. Try berberine supplementation (see page 112).
4. Eat a low-FODMAP diet (see page 180).
5. Consider taking out all grains and beans from your diet.
6. Get a breath test to identify small intestinal bacterial overgrowth (SIBO; see page 182).

HOW REINTRODUCTION WORKS

If you've determined that you're ready to begin reintroducing foods, let me explain to you a little more about the process.

After two weeks of phases 1 and 2, your system should be very calm, which will make it very clear to you when you introduce a food that doesn't agree with your system. When you reintroduce foods, you are challenging or testing trigger foods to see if you have a reaction. You are acting like a diet detective, searching for the source of your symptoms.

To challenge a food, you will eat the food two to three times a day for three days in a row. If at any time during the three-day period you notice a change in the way you feel, then you will remove the food from your diet and wait until your symptoms completely disappear before challenging the next food (this could take a few days or a week or more).

DON'T GIVE IN TO DENIAL

A common mistake is to write off the connection between foods and symptoms, in spite of the evidence. Many of my clients will work hard to convince themselves that it is not the food bringing their symptoms back. They're so accustomed to thinking that it has to be something else that once made them feel similar symptoms. For example:

- "My fatigue is probably just because I didn't sleep well last night."
- "This congestion and nasal drip must be from a cold that is coming on."
- "I wonder if this joint pain is from all the gardening or exercise yesterday?"

If you have faithfully followed the phases of the program and the reintroduction of a food produces your symptoms, the food is most likely the cause. Here is the tried-and-true rule that has saved many of my clients months of time in doing another elimination diet: "When in doubt... leave it out!" The minute you notice the symptom, stop eating that food.

You *must* let your system return to a state of calm before testing another food, or you'll risk inaccurate results. For example, if you have a reaction to dairy and you test gluten too soon after, your conclusion might be that you're sensitive to both when really it could just be the dairy. If you cut corners here, you will risk landing right back into the same pool of symptoms with no clear answer to the cause. Being patient will prevent unnecessary long-term dietary restrictions.

Even if you don't have a noticeable reaction, you must challenge only one food at a time to ensure accurate results. If a food does not cause a reaction during reintroduction, it is safe to keep in your diet for the rest of the program.

If a food causes a reaction, it should be kept out of your diet for at least three months before challenging it again. Remember to keep detailed journal entries of the Reintroduction phase, documenting times, dates, and specific physical or emotional responses (see page 97 for more on how to keep a diet journal). Here's a list of potential reactions to reintroduced foods:

- Fatigue, lethargy, feeling like you're "walking through molasses"
- Foggy thinking, memory issues, feeling like you're "not as sharp as usual," lack of focus
- Moodiness, anxiety, depression, aggression, hyperactivity, racing thoughts, insomnia
- Bowel changes, gas, diarrhea, constipation, bloating, reflux (GERD), cramping
- Muscle pain, joint pain, back and neck pain
- Headaches, migraines
- Runny nose, sinus congestion, coughing, asthma
- Rashes, eczema, psoriasis, flushing, hives
- Heart palpitations, rapid pulse, rapid breathing
- Nausea, vomiting
- Numbness, tingling

YOUR REINTRODUCTION SCHEDULE

To make it easy to follow this program, here is a proposed schedule you can use to reintroduce foods. This schedule may vary depending on your food choices or known allergens. We recommend that you wait as long as possible to reintroduce dairy, gluten, soy, and corn, as many people react to these foods. They also tend to cause strong reactions, so that it may take a while (possibly weeks) for symptoms to subside before you can continue adding other foods back in. Make sure to track all of your symptoms in your Elimination Diet Journal; see page 98 for an example, or download a free printable PDF from our website, WholeLifeNutrition.net.

You'll notice specific days listed next to the foods—for example, citrus is suggested to be tested on days 15 to 17. These days are meant to be a guideline only. If you have a reaction to a particular food or foods and need to wait until reintroducing the next food, the calendar will shift. Also, if you see a food listed that isn't part of your normal diet, don't feel the need to test it just because it's listed here. Simply skip that food and move on to the next. And remember that once you've tested a food and it's proven okay for you—that is, it didn't trigger a reaction—you can leave it in and continue to test other foods.

We've included suggested foods and recipes to try when you reintroduce each food. Starting on page 172, you'll also find suggested sample days with what to eat for each meal.

It's recommended that you wait to challenge **alcohol**, **coffee**, and **black tea** until all of the previous foods have been reintroduced.

If you decide to add them in earlier, be sure to choose gluten-free alcohols and leave cream and sugar out until they are properly challenged.

1. **Citrus:** Add freshly squeezed lemon and lime juice to smoothies and fresh juices for the first day of the citrus challenge; on the second and third day, all citrus is fair game so add items like oranges, tangerines, and mandarins. (It is really important to make sure your citrus is organic; otherwise, there may be chemicals on and in the citrus that will cause reactions.) (Days 15 to 17)
2. **Nightshade Vegetables:** Make mashed potatoes; add diced potatoes to chicken soup; add bell peppers to stir-fries and soups; make a tomato-based marinara sauce and serve it over rice noodles or spaghetti squash; add eggplant to stews; snack on goji berries; use curry powder, chili powder, chipotle chile powder, and paprika now in your cooking. (Days 18 to 20)

NIGHTSHADE WATCH

Some people can react to one variety of nightshade vegetable and not another. If you've noticed an obvious connection between eating tomatoes, peppers, or eggplant and a flare-up of your symptoms in the past, it would be best to challenge each separately for three days. If you have not observed an obvious connection between nightshades and your symptoms, just test all nightshades as one group.

---

3. **Beef:** Make the Nightshade-Free Beef Stew (page 220), prepare organic grass-fed steak, add ground beef to sauces or make burgers, make beef bone broths. (Days 21 to 23)

4. **Pork:** Avoid bacon, sausages, or ham because of additives that can cause potential reactions; make slow-cooked pulled pork or pork chops, or make homemade sausage patties using ground organic pork and fresh sage. (Days 24 to 26)

5. **Sesame:** Use organic tahini in salad dressings; or add sesame seeds to salads or stir-fries. (Days 27 to 29)

6. **Walnuts and Pecans:** Toast raw walnuts and pecans in the oven for 15 minutes at 375°F and add them to fresh salads or Coconut-Quinoa Breakfast Porridge (page 198). (Days 30 to 32)

7. **Almonds:** Eat organic almond butter with apple slices; soak raw almonds overnight to make Raw Vanilla Almond Milk (page 290) or to add to smoothies. (Days 33 to 35)

8. **Cashews:** Use raw cashew butter and raw cashews in smoothies and desserts; try the Pumpkin Pie Chia Pudding (page 286). (Days 36 to 38)

9. **Peanuts:** Use organic dry-roasted peanuts or fresh shelled peanuts and eat plain as a snack, or eat apple slices dipped in organic roasted peanut butter. (Days 39 to 41)

10. **Hazelnuts, Pistachios, Brazil Nuts, and Macadamia Nuts:** Eat organic nuts as snacks or add to salads or meals. (Days 42 to 44)

11. **Sugar:** Use organic cane sugar in baking in place of coconut sugar, or added to herbal tea. (Days 45 to 47)

12. **Chocolate:** Use raw cacao powder or cacao nibs and add to smoothies or make Chocolate Zucchini Cupcakes (page 285). (Days 48 to 50)

13. **Corn:** Use fresh organic corn on the cob or organic frozen corn kernels. (Days 51 to 53)

14. **Soy:** Use organic wheat-free tamari, tofu, and tempeh. (Days 54 to 56)

15. **Yeast:** Add nutritional yeast to salads, soups, and sprinkle on main dishes; use baker's yeast and make gluten-free rice bread (see page 227); and use other organic vinegars such as balsamic and red wine vinegar. (Days 57 to 59)

16. **Eggs:** Pastured and organic is ideal—make scrambled, hard-boiled eggs or baked into muffins—try the Sweet Potato Spice Muffins (page 227). (Days 60 to 62)

When you are ready to test the following foods that are more likely to cause a reaction, wait until at least day 50 and follow these guidelines:

17. **Dairy:** Use plain organic yogurt, organic raw whole milk or cream, and organic sour cream. (Days 63 to 65)
18. **Gluten:** Use organic sourdough rye bread (French Meadow Bakery makes one that you can purchase in the frozen section of your local health food store) or pearled barley. (Days 66 to 68)
19. **Wheat:** Use organic whole wheat berries and flour to test for wheat; add in other gluten-free grains and lentils once you have challenged gluten. (Days 69 to 71)

NOTE: Some people may have reactions to wheat but not to gluten. By testing the gluten reactions with rye and barley first, you can determine if you react to both.

> Wait to challenge **alcohol**, **coffee**, and **black tea** until all of the previous foods have been reintroduced.

PHASE 3: REINTRODUCTION MEAL PLANS AND RECIPE LIST

As you prepare to reintroduce foods, use these sample days to plan your meals. Revisit these at least a couple of days before you're set to test each food. Make sure you're stocked with all the ingredients you need to make the appropriate recipes for each challenge food. Remember that you will be challenging these foods over a three-day period, so get creative with your menu plans.

Citrus

Breakfast: Very Berry Chia Smoothie, with the juice of 1 to 2 lemons or limes added (page 192)
Lunch: Raw Kale Salad with Lemon and Garlic (page 235) with sautéed organic chicken breast or cooked wild salmon
Snack: Avocado-Mint Mini Tarts (page 283)
Dinner: Black Bean, Yam, and Avocado Tacos (page 255), served with lime wedges

Nightshade Vegetables

Breakfast: Sweet Potato–Kale Hash with variation (page 200)

Lunch: Summer Vegetable Soup (page 215)

Snack: carrot sticks, red bell pepper slices, sprouted pumpkin seeds

Dinner: Whole Roasted Chicken with Rosemary (page 265), baked potatoes, steamed green beans, organic baby green salad greens with Creamy Sunflower Seed–Parsley Dressing (page 275)

Beef

Breakfast: Turkey, Kale, and Carrot Hash (page 199) made with ground beef instead of turkey

Lunch: Roasted Delicata Squash Salad with Apples and Toasted Pumpkin Seeds (page 231) topped with leftover cooked salmon or sliced grilled steak

Snack: Green Cleansing Juice (page 190)

Dinner: Nightshade-Free Beef Stew (page 220)

Pork

Breakfast: 2 organic pork breakfast sausages, 2 cups Strawberry-Kale-Mint Smoothie (page 194)

Lunch: Mung Bean, Zucchini, and Dill Soup (page 211)

Snack: apple slices and pumpkin seed butter

Dinner: organic pork chops, whipped sweet potatoes, steamed green beans

Sesame

Breakfast: 2 to 3 cups Ginger-Berry Smoothie (page 192)

Lunch: Adzuki Bean and Rice Salad (page 248) made with cold-pressed sesame oil and topped with toasted sesame seeds

Snack: Hummus (homemade only, page 271) made with tahini and fresh carrots

Dinner: Vegetable Chicken Bake (page 263), Raw Kale Salad with Lemon and Garlic (page 235) sprinkled with toasted sesame seeds, Roasted Root Vegetables (page 241)

Walnuts and Pecans

Breakfast: Coconut-Quinoa Breakfast Porridge (page 198) topped with chopped raw pecans

Lunch: Turkey Vegetable Soup (page 217)

Snack: handful of raw walnuts and a few Medjool dates

Dinner: Herb-Roasted Wild Salmon (page 257), Roasted Delicata Squash Salad with Apples and Toasted Pumpkin Seeds (page 231) topped with lightly roasted raw walnuts or pecans

Almonds

Breakfast: Strawberry-Almond Milkshake (page 196), Coconut-Quinoa Breakfast Porridge (page 198)

Lunch: Mustard-Herb Lamb Burger (page 270) wrapped in a lettuce leaf with cucumber slices, fresh mint leaves, and a dollop of Coconut Sour Cream (page 277)

Snack: Almond Butter Cookies (page 284) or apples dipped in roasted almond butter

Dinner: Turkey Vegetable Soup (page 217), salad made of leaf lettuce, grated carrots, roasted almonds, and Fresh Broccoli Sprouts (page 301) along with your favorite Elimination Diet salad dressing (pages 271 to 276)

Cashews

Breakfast: Creamy Rice Cereal (page 198) topped with fresh berries and Vanilla Cashew Milk (page 291)

Lunch: Greek Chicken Lettuce Wraps (page 267)

Snack: handful of raw cashews, fresh organic raspberries

Dinner: Baked Salmon with Cashew-Ginger Sauce (page 258) served with baked sweet potatoes and sautéed kale

Peanuts

Breakfast: Banana Muffin (page 225) spread with 2 tablespoons organic peanut butter (only ingredients should be peanuts and sea salt), 2 cups Pineapple Green Smoothie (page 194)

Lunch: Turkey, Kale, and Carrot Hash (page 199)

Snack: 2 handfuls of organic dry-roasted peanuts

Dinner: Sautéed organic chicken breasts, baked sweet potatoes, Grated Raw Vegetable Bliss Salad (page 229) topped with crushed, roasted organic peanuts

Sugar

Breakfast: Creamy Rice Cereal (page 198) sprinkled with organic cane sugar or organic brown sugar

Lunch: simple green salad with leftover roasted chicken or salmon and your favorite Elimination Diet salad dressing (pages 271 to 276)

Snack: Banana Muffin (page 225) made with organic cane sugar instead of coconut sugar

Dinner: 2 chopped chicken breasts marinated in a sauce made from a few tablespoons coconut aminos, juice of ½ lime, 2 tablespoons organic cane sugar, fresh ginger and garlic, then sautéed in coconut oil. Serve with sautéed broccoli, onions, and bok choy over a bed of white or brown rice.

Chocolate

Breakfast: smoothie made from soaked raw almonds or raw cashews, water, frozen bananas, and raw cacao powder

Lunch: Turkey, Kale, and Carrot Hash (page 199)

Snack: Chocolate Zucchini Cupcake (page 285)

Dinner: Chicken Vegetable Soup (page 216)

Yeast

Breakfast: slice of Chia-Rice Sandwich Bread (page 227) spread with pumpkin seed butter or almond butter, 1 small banana

Lunch: sandwich made from 2 slices Chia-Rice Sandwich Bread (page 227), organic turkey slices, mashed avocado, organic Dijon mustard, and lettuce leaves

Snack: 1 to 2 cups Carrot-Cucumber-Ginger Juice (page 190)

Dinner: Herb-Roasted Wild Salmon (page 257), baked sweet potatoes, large green salad served with a balsamic dressing (¼ cup extra-virgin olive oil, 3 tablespoons organic balsamic vinegar, 2 to 3 teaspoons pure maple syrup, 1 teaspoon organic Dijon mustard, ¼ teaspoon sea salt)

Eggs

Breakfast: Kale, Zucchini, and Egg Scramble (page 203), Celeriac-Rutabaga Hash Browns (page 203), few spoonfuls of Rainbow Kraut (page 299)

Lunch: 2 hardboiled eggs with a green salad and your favorite Elimination Diet salad dressing (pages 271 to 276)

Snack: 1 Sweet Potato Spice Muffin (page 227)

Dinner: Mung Bean, Zucchini, and Dill Soup (page 211)

PHASE 3 RECIPES

In the recipe chapter (page 189), you'll find several other recipes that you can try during phase 3. Here's the complete list:

Ginger-Berry Smoothie

Berry Vanilla Milkshake

Strawberry-Almond Milkshake

Chocolate-Avocado Milkshake

Kale, Zucchini, and Egg Scramble

Mung Bean, Zucchini, and Dill Soup

Summer Vegetable Soup

Nightshade-Free Beef Stew

Almond Flour Tortillas

Carrot Breakfast Muffins

Sweet Potato Spice Muffins

Chia-Rice Sandwich Bread

Grated Raw Vegetable Bliss Salad

Raw Kale Salad with Lemon and Garlic

Raw Cauliflower, Lemon, and Leek Salad

Quinoa-Cucumber-Dill Salad

Chickpea Curry with Potatoes and Kale

Poached Salmon with Summer Vegetables

Baked Salmon with Cashew-Ginger Sauce

Greek Chicken Lettuce Wraps

Hummus

Lemon-Garlic Dressing

Cashew Ranch Dressing

Avocado-Mint Mini Tarts

Almond Butter Cookies

Chocolate Zucchini Cupcakes

Pumpkin Pie Chia Pudding

Raw Vanilla Almond Milk

Vanilla Cashew Milk

WHEN YOUR COMFORT FOOD IS DISCOMFORT FOOD

Some of our favorite comfort foods contain the top trigger foods. Mac and cheese, bread with butter, peanut butter and jelly sandwiches, ice cream, cookies fresh out of the oven, coffee, potato chips, doughnuts, mashed potatoes... they're all loaded with some of the most common irritants. What do you do if your dietary detective work has revealed these foods are not the source of your comfort, but the cause of your discomfort?

Many of my clients are disappointed when they discover that their favorite foods don't agree with them, but this is often balanced with the fact that they feel so much better by the time they figure this out. In many ways, it's a relief to finally know the cause of the weight gain, mind fog, aches, and pains. And this empowering knowledge—that eliminating these foods will give them a new, healthier life—is enough motivation to keep them from truly missing those old, harmful favorites. When faced with the choice, "Do I want the suffering or do I want the foods?" they choose to pass on the foods.

If your reactions aren't that bad, you might wonder: What's the harm in indulging in problem foods every so often? I would warn you that even "mild" symptoms of skin flare-ups, bowel changes, mild fatigue, and sinus congestion indicate that your body is under attack by inflammatory signals. This background inflammation will leave you more susceptible for most diseases. The longer you consume foods that irritate your intestines and your body, the more likely you are to promote autoimmune and other diseases.

In people who react to gluten, small exposures can mean big problems. A 2001 article in *Lancet* authored by researchers with the University of Milano-Bicocca in Italy showed that people who had celiac disease and were not really strict in avoiding gluten were 600 percent more likely to die from a disease over a 30-year period compared to their counterparts who were very strict.

Additional research published in the *Journal of the American Medical Association* in 2009 by Dr. Jonas Ludvigsson and others echoed this finding, adding concern for those individuals with gluten intolerance as well. They found a:

- 39 percent increased risk of death in celiacs who cheated on their diet
- 35 percent increased risk of death in those with gluten sensitivity
- 72 percent increased risk of death in those who had intestinal inflammation related to gluten consumption

In my personal experience with food reactions, I fought the truth for a while. I would eat burritos with a whole-wheat tortilla and think, "It's whole wheat; it should be good for me! How could a whole food be bad for me?" Or I would often think: "Maybe I've grown out of it by now?" And yet every single time I ate gluten, diarrhea, joint pain, fatigue, and a foul mood would follow within 2 to 24 hours. It was like a hangover after a fun night out. As I got older, the pain and suffering worsened and I began to wonder...is it really worth it? I finally realized that eating the foods that irritated me was like banging my head against the wall and then wondering why my head hurt so much. It had to stop.

If the Elimination Diet reveals that you have food reactions, it's completely natural to feel trapped and overwhelmed by it at first. But you should know that this feeling is only temporary—there is a brand new world out there for you, one filled with fantastic recipes, restaurants, and experiences.

Be sure to use all the wonderful recipes in this book and visit our community online to exchange ideas and share experiences with others. I used to curse my food sensitivities for limiting me so much socially. Now, I bless them for forcing me to find healthier foods that have brought my life to a completely new and incredible level. And along the way, I have been able to help thousands of other people reduce their suffering.

10

FREQUENTLY ASKED QUESTIONS AND SPECIAL CONSIDERATIONS

After using the Elimination Diet for more than a decade to help people of all ages, backgrounds, and symptoms, I've encountered just about every question and issue there is. Hopefully, the answers provided here will help you make modifications or resolve any issues. If you're still stumped, reach out to our website, WholeLifeNutrition.net, for our Elimination Diet resources.

Is it normal to have intense cravings for cheese, bread, sugar, and caffeine that border on drug-like addiction?

Yes, especially if you have a history of addiction in your family. There are compounds found in these foods or produced after consuming these foods that can have drug-like effects on your body. Cheese, interestingly enough, appears to be the worst offender. I have had clients dream about cheese, draw pictures of cheese, get anxious without cheese, get the shakes without cheese . . . it is really surprising how powerful cheese cravings can be.

But you don't have to white-knuckle it along. Having a high concentration of antioxidant- and detoxification-supporting foods like broccoli sprouts, kale, and radishes can help. So can Epsom salt baths and supplementing with a high-quality multivitamin.

My best advice if you're having cravings is to hang in there. Symptoms are usually worse in the first four to six days and get better soon after that. If your caffeine headaches are unbearable, you may want to wean yourself off with green tea (see page 131).

I am experiencing more gas than usual during the first few days of the diet. Is this normal?

Yes, this is normal for some people. As the gut detoxes, gut microflora changes. Your body may take some time to adjust.

For some people, especially those with severely damaged guts, the gas and bloating could be caused by bacterial imbalances, fructose intolerance, gastric acid insufficiency, or a pancreatic enzyme deficiency. We recommend removing apples, pears, dates, beans, cherries, watermelon, asparagus, avocados, garlic, onions, and cauliflower for a period of time to see if your symptoms improve. If your symptoms persist, see the recommendations below.

When it comes to fruits and gas, FODMAP avoidance is key. See the next question for more on FODMAPs.

What is the FODMAP diet and do I need to follow it?

FODMAP stands for fermentable oligosaccharides, disaccharides, monosaccharides, and polylols. These are all forms of carbohydrates that are more readily fermented by bacteria. Easily fermented carbohydrates have been shown to contribute to SIBO.

If you have gas, bloating, diarrhea, or "gooey poops" after you eat pears or drink apple juice, you can first try to reduce the quantity of fruit smoothies you are drinking at any given time. If you are drinking 16 ounces now, cut that amount in half to 8 ounces and see if that helps. The next step is to take out foods high in FODMAPs for a while and see how you feel.

FODMAP reactions are most often temporary and will go away once your intestinal flora have been balanced out. Reactions usually occur when you eat too many foods rich in fermentable carbohydrates at one sitting. For example, you might tolerate a quarter of an apple before having a reaction, whereas half of an apple might bring back the bloating.

Here is a list of common foods on our program that have FODMAPs in them. These are to be avoided if you have symptoms of bloating, gas, nausea, diarrhea, and/or constipation that are persisting. (Note: You will have already eliminated some of these foods during the Elimination Diet):

Vegetables: onions, cauliflower, beets (root), asparagus, garlic, sweet potatoes, mushrooms

Fruits: apples, avocados, mangoes, pears, watermelon, nectarines, apricots, blackberries, cherries

Grains: quinoa, brown rice and rice flour, white jasmine rice, rice noodles, and quinoa pasta (corn-free) are okay to eat. The highest FODMAP grain is wheat. Other grains that include high levels of FODMAPs are rye, barley, and spelt. Note that none of the grains used in this Elimination Diet program contain FODMAPs, so they are okay to eat if you suspect a FODMAP sensitivity.

Legumes: garbanzo beans, black beans, adzuki beans, more than ½ cup lima beans

Nuts: almonds, cashews, pistachios

Dairy: Lactose from dairy products is a high-FODMAP food.

You can also download the FODMAP app from researchers at Monash University in Australia, where the FODMAP diet was created. It's available online at www.med.monash.edu/cecs/gastro/fodmap.

What is Starch Maldigestion and what can I do about it?

Foods such as potatoes, whole grains, and legumes contain long chains of sugars in them called starches. Our intestinal cells can only absorb single sugars so our bodies have to break these chains apart before we can absorb and use them. Proteins called enzymes secreted from our saliva and pancreas break the bonds in the chains of sugars until small pairs of two sugar molecules called disaccharides are left. The last and possibly most important step of breaking these into single sugars is left to enzymes located in the wall of the intestines. Problems arise when these intestinal enzymes can't do their job. Many things that irritate the intestines or leave it susceptible to damage, such as food sensitivity reactions, toxins, bacteria, parasites, stress, and poor nutrition can impede the activity of these enzymes. Interestingly, there are some populations that have less production of these disaccharidase enzymes to begin with. For example, a 2011 article in the journal *PLoS One* demonstrated that autistic children were more likely to have lower disaccharidase levels in the intestines and an imbalance in bacteria as well. Without this enzyme activity that frees up the sugars for absorption into the body, these pairs of sugars (dissacharides) get digested and consumed by local bacteria. The bacteria can then overgrow, leading to further irritation of the intestinal wall. These undigested particles can also cause a release of fluid from the intestines as an attempt to flush them out. The resulting symptoms people can experience include gas, nausea, bloating, cramping, and diarrhea. Starch maldigestion may eventually then lead to SIBO (see below).

If you experience these symptoms, or have the diagnosis of inflammatory bowel disease (Crohn's and ulcerative colitis) or irritable bowel syndrome, you may benefit from doing an elimination diet that excludes all complex starches.

To modify the elimination diet for starch maldigestion, remove all whole grains (brown rice, white rice, wild rice, quinoa, whole grain flours) and all legumes. Additionally, you must remove other complex starches such as sweet potatoes and yams, maple syrup, tapioca flour, arrowroot powder, seaweeds, flaxseeds, and chia seeds. Your diet will consist of animal proteins, fats, vegetables, fruits, seeds (pumpkin and sunflower), and small amounts of raw honey and dates to allow the intestines to fully heal. After the gut is totally calm you can enter Phase 3 and begin to challenge foods. Keep out sugar, corn, soy, yeast, dairy, and gluten until the very end of the Phase 3. All other challenge foods are safe for someone following the starch maldigestion variation.

What is SIBO (Small Intestinal Bacterial Overgrowth) and what can I do about it?

More and more people are suffering from distention and bloating after eating. This can be a sign of having an overgrowth of bacteria in your small intestines. Partner those symptoms with nausea, cramping, diarrhea, constipation, or alternating diarrhea and constipation that persists for over three months, and chances are quite high that you may have SIBO.

Normally, the upper intestinal tract has very little bacteria in it compared to the lower intestines. While the colon is a cauldron of bacteria teaming with trillions upon trillions of organisms, the upper intestinal tract is relatively vacant in comparison. There are multiple things that assure that this area is kept clear of too many organisms.

Adequate digestion of food by stomach acid, pancreatic enzymes, and intestinal "brush border" enzymes allow food to be in small particles that are easily absorbed by the body. If the foods are not digested properly, they can be consumed by bacteria and contribute to their colonization and growth in the upper intestinal tract.

Muscle contractions called the *migrating motor complex* squeeze the contents of the upper intestines and force them to travel along toward the lower intestines. This sweeps out undigested food and bacteria in the upper intestines approximately 4 hours after food is eaten.

Vitamin D assists intestinal cells in secreting their own version of antibiotics called antimicrobial peptides that kill off harmful bacteria that try to colonize along the intestinal surface. Healthy intestinal cells also secrete immunoglobulins (immune system antibodies) that attach to bacteria and stop them from causing harm.

When a person has low stomach acid, low pancreatic enzyme and bile secretions, poor secretion of protective immunoglobulins from intestinal cells, low migrating motor complex function, and low vitamin D, they are more likely to have undigested food in the upper intestinal tract and SIBO. Add in damage to the intestinal tract by toxins, a poor diet, stress, and nutrient deficiencies, and SIBO can become severe.

There are a few things you can do to help you turn the corner and most of them have already been mentioned in this book.

1. Find the foods that are irritating your intestines by doing the elimination diet.
2. Check your gastric acid secretion and use a betaine HCL supplement with meals if it is low.
3. Look for signs of fat malabsorption and take digestive enzymes if necessary.
4. Leave adequate time between meals (approximately 4 hours) unless you have been diagnosed with hypoglycemia.
5. Check your vitamin D levels and start supplementation if necessary.
6. Eating recipes rich in mushrooms appears to increase immunoglobulin A (IgA) from the intestinal cells, which has been shown to keep bacteria from entering the intestinal lining, thereby protecting the gut wall from damage.

To modify the elimination diet for SIBO, follow the starch maldigestion and low-FODMAP variations mentioned previously. When severe, SIBO can require intense interventions. Treatment options for SIBO include antimicrobial herbs (high dose garlic and berberine), elemental diets, and antibiotics. For proper testing and treatments for SIBO, go to SIBOinfo.com.

I really can't have coffee or tea on the diet?

I'm afraid not. No coffee is allowed, only herbal teas. Try chamomile, mint, ginger, raspberry leaf, and nettle teas. You can add back coffee and other teas at the end of Phase 3: Reintroduction. Caffeine is a stimulant and affects liver detoxification.

Some people get terrible caffeine headaches, cravings, and irritability that are so bad they discontinue the diet. If you are finding your caffeine withdrawal to be unbearable, have a cup of green or white tea. You can add a little honey if you like for an extra antioxidant and immune-boosting combination.

If you reuse the tea bag for a second cup, you will get even more anti-oxidants and less caffeine. Make sure you drink plenty of fluids, eat broccoli sprouts, take Epsom salt baths, and have some activated charcoal on hand to lessen these symptoms.

What about herbs and spices—can I have those?

Yes, you can have dried herbs and spices that are gluten-free, additive-free, and preservative-free. Please check with the manufacturer to make sure they are processed in a gluten-free facility. As was mentioned earlier, we highly recommend organic spices. Of course, all fresh herbs are in.

When can I add regular vinegar? I don't see it on the list.

Keep all vinegars, except for raw organic apple cider vinegar and coconut vinegar, out of your diet until after you challenge yeast in Phase 3: Reintro-duction. Vinegar contains yeast and this is why we keep it out until the end of the diet. Raw organic cider vinegar and coconut vinegar seem to be toler-ated by most.

Fermented foods like vinegar may contribute to headaches and/or anxi-ety in some people with sensitivities to amines.

When can I add vanilla?

Add alcohol-extracted vanilla during the reintroduction phase when you challenge alcohol. Non-alcoholic vanilla can be used during all phases. We prefer to use raw organic vanilla powder in many recipes, which is suitable for all phases.

I get a headache every time I eat sauerkraut and fermented vegetables. Why?

Fermented foods are high in histamine, which can contribute to headaches, anxiety, or even aggression in some susceptible individuals. If you notice a pattern in your food journal with some of these symptoms and fermented vegetable consumption or vinegars, then omit them from your diet.

I find that sometimes I can tolerate a certain food while other times I cannot. Can you explain?

Sometimes we are able to tolerate only a small amount of a particular food with no reaction. Other times you consume that food you may eat more than your body can handle and so you will have a reaction. Another reason for varying responses to food has to do with what's going on in the intestines at the time of eating the food. If your intestines are calm, your microbes are balanced, and you have plenty nutrients around to lessen your immune response (vitamin D, essential fatty acids, Meriva, etc. . . .), a food may be less troublesome. If any of those factors are out of balance in that moment, you are more likely to have a reaction. As you read in Part 1 of this book, environmental toxins may throw off many of these factors.

Is this an anti-candida diet?

No. Although this Elimination Diet will assist in lowering the growth of the troublesome yeast known as *Candida albicans*, it was not designed with that intention in mind. *Candida albicans* thrives in an intestinal environment lacking in beneficial microbes and vegetables and full of junk food. The Elimination Diet is far from that.

Can I drink kombucha on the diet?

No, although kombucha may be well tolerated and beneficial to health for most people, some individuals may not react well to the yeasts. Additionally, depending on many factors, some of the sugar and caffeine may still be present in the brew. Wait to add kombucha back into your diet until after you have challenged yeast and cane sugar.

What if I want to cheat?

Cheating will drastically affect your results. I had the privilege to interview world-renowned gastroenterologist Alessio Fasano in 2013. During the interview, he said "100 percent effort equals 100 percent results. Ninety-nine percent effort equals 0 percent results!" Unfortunately for would-be cheaters, the tiniest bit of irritating food can set off your immune system for weeks. And this makes perfect sense. Your immune system is designed to react to minute bacteria and viruses. Once you are exposed to them, your immune cells will stay excited in case they need to continue battling them. This will make it impossible to pinpoint the full list of foods that works and doesn't work for your unique body chemistry. Long story short: Cheating will completely change your results of the Elimination Diet.

Why do you leave out agave?

When fructose is eaten with a similar amount of glucose as is common in most natural foods, both of the sugars are fairly well absorbed. When the ratio of fructose is much higher, the fructose is not well absorbed and can lead to symptoms of gas, bloating, and diarrhea. Agave is very high in fructose (between 60 and 90 percent of the sugar in agave is fructose), unlike other sugars that have a more balanced ratio of fructose to glucose.

Can I put my child on the Elimination Diet?

Children who are having problems with attention disorders, eczema, stomach upset, asthma, ear infections, and keeping weight on can benefit greatly from this program. The most important aspect of making this diet work for children is to make sure they are eating enough.

To do this, skip phase 1—the two-day detox—and move right into phase 2. Foods featured in the Detox Phase can still be consumed, but should be eaten in balance with other foods. For example, your child can still enjoy the green smoothies from phase 1; I just do not advise that they fast on them. Follow phase 2 for a full fourteen days.

For children with less severe issues, such as mild cases of eczema, asthma, or bowel problems, it is possible to modify the diet further to make it simpler and easier to follow. Since you'll be starting with the Elimination Phase, you'll want to focus on getting all the processed foods out of the diet as well as removing all sources of gluten, dairy, eggs, corn, soy, and yeast. You can keep in nightshade vegetables, nuts, and some citrus (only lemons and limes), as well as sesame, beef, and pork (make sure it is pastured/organic).

If your child does not respond to this and is still having gut-related issues, then remove all grains, legumes, and starchy vegetables from the diet (potatoes, sweet potatoes, yams). Make sure you are supplementing with digestive enzymes and a high-quality probiotic (see Resources on page 303 for recommendations).

Can I do the diet while pregnant?

Yes, absolutely. The key to following the Elimination Diet during pregnancy is to make sure you are consuming enough calories. As a result, you may want to do a less restrictive version of the Elimination Diet that allows you to keep in some common calorie-dense foods. Keeping in access to all nuts, seeds, pork, beef, nightshade vegetables, and citrus will assist you in meeting these needs.

Doing the Elimination Diet during pregnancy can have a tremendous benefit for your unborn baby. If your gut is being affected by an unknown food sensitivity, then you might not be able to absorb all of the key nutrients needed for growing a healthy baby. Both calming the gut and discovering your food sensitivities are key.

To modify the Elimination Diet for pregnancy, we recommend skipping the restrictive two-day detox (phase 1) and jumping right into phase 2. But since the phase 1 recipes are incredibly healing and nutritionally dense, include all of the phase 1 recipes in your diet during the entire program.

All of the recipes in this book are full of the key nutrients needed for a healthy pregnancy, so know that by going on this diet you are giving your unborn baby a tremendous gift of health right from the start.

Please note that it can be extremely difficult to follow the Elimination Diet during pregnancy if you are vegan or vegetarian—this is likely to limit dietary choices too much and may put your baby at risk for not getting adequate nutrients. If you are vegetarian or vegan, you may want to try a gluten-free and dairy-free (if you are not already vegan) diet during this time instead, and supplement with calcium and vitamin D.

Can I do the diet during lactation?

Many lactating mothers choose to follow an elimination diet if their breast-fed baby is experiencing chronic colic, reflux, skin irritations like eczema, as well as ear infections. If a mother's gut is out of balance and leaky, large food proteins can pass through undigested into her breast milk.

To modify the Elimination Diet for lactation, skip the first two-day detox (phase 1) and jump right into phase 2. Incorporate phase 1 recipes into your daily meals. Keeping in access to all nuts, seeds, pork, beef, and nightshade vegetables while breast-feeding will help you meet the extra calorie demands while on the Elimination Diet.

However, you may need to modify our diet even further and avoid things like raw garlic in salad dressings and raw kale and other cruciferous vegetables if your baby is very gassy.

All babies are different—some thrive off breast milk from moms who consume raw garlic, broccoli, and dairy products while other babies can get very irritated. Here are some foods that can irritate a newborn baby and cause colic:

- Dairy
- Raw garlic and onions
- Raw cruciferous vegetables (broccoli, cauliflower, Brussels sprouts, kale, collards)
- Citrus, especially oranges and grapefruit
- Peanuts
- Chocolate
- Caffeine
- Spicy peppers

The best way to determine what's upsetting your baby is to follow an elimination diet with the modifications listed. Be sure to journal or document how your baby responds to foods as you reintroduce them to your diet.

I'm an athlete—will this diet provide enough nutrients and calories?

Absolutely. Ultramarathon runners, Crossfit competitors, and other extreme athletes have completed the Elimination Diet. Just make sure you are eating an adequate amount of calories while on the program. This may mean eating lots of extra snacks, and larger meals to accommodate your needs.

11

RECIPES

Welcome to the Elimination Diet recipes. These will be the delicious tools for healing your symptoms and changing your life! Here you'll find recipes to suit all eating styles and variations of the diet.

A few notes before you dig in:

- All of the recipes are noted for specific phases. If you are in phase 1 just stick with all of the recipes that have this phase 1 icon in the recipe: `Phase 1`. However, if you are in phase 2, you can enjoy both phase 1 and phase 2 recipes. Look for recipes with this symbol for phase 2 recipes: `Phase 2`. And in phase 3 of the diet, you will be able to enjoy all of the recipes that say phase 1 and phase 2. Look for recipes with this symbol for phase 3 recipes: `Phase 3`.
- There are also variations included in many of the recipes, which will make them work for other phases of the diet. For example, a recipe may be noted as phase 2, but can be adapted to be used in phase 3 for challenging certain foods.
- Watch for the low-FODMAP symbol to indicate which recipes will be best for you if you are following the low-FODMAP variation of the diet. `Low FODMAP`

For more Elimination Diet recipes, please be sure to check out *The Whole Life Nutrition Cookbook* and our Nourishing Meals recipe blog at Nourishing Meals.com.

CARROT-CUCUMBER-GINGER JUICE

Phase 1 *Detox*

Low FODMAP

Use this recipe during the two-day detox as well as throughout the entire diet.

6 large carrots	1 (2-inch) piece fresh ginger
3 medium cucumbers	

Place all the ingredients into the feed tube of your juicer. Juice according to the manufacturer's directions. Pour the fresh juice into a glass and enjoy immediately.

Yield: about 3 cups

GREEN CLEANSING JUICE

Phase 1 *Detox*

We make some variation of this juice a few times a week! Get creative and add whatever vegetables you want. If the flavor is too strong, just add one chopped Granny Smith apple to the mix and it will slightly sweeten the juice.

4 to 5 celery stalks	1 to 2 cups chopped fresh pineapple
2 medium cucumbers	2 black kale leaves
1 to 2 cups chopped green cabbage	1 (1-inch) piece fresh ginger

Place all the ingredients into the feed tube of your juicer. Juice according to the manufacturer's directions. Pour the fresh juice into a glass and enjoy immediately.

Yield: about 2½ cups

PURPLE VEGETABLE JUICE

Phase 1 *Detox*

You will feel refreshed after drinking this juice; plus, cabbage juice is an excellent stomach tonic. Once you have reintroduced citrus, try adding a whole peeled Meyer lemon (or regular lemon) to the juice—it elevates the flavors to the next level!

¼ head red cabbage	½ Granny Smith apple
2 medium cucumbers	1 (1-inch) piece fresh ginger
3 to 4 celery stalks	

Place all the ingredients into the feed tube of your juicer. Juice according to the manufacturer's directions. Pour the fresh juice into a glass and enjoy immediately.

Yield: about 2 cups

BEET-FENNEL JUICE

Phase 1 *Detox*

This is one of my favorite juice recipes. I've been drinking it ever since I started going to juice bars and ordering custom-made juice blends. The fennel adds a nice sweet flavor—it feels like a treat to me! I use the whole fennel bulb—the white portion, green stalks, and feathery leaves.

1 whole fennel bulb, cut into pieces	1 ripe pear, quartered
1 small beet, quartered	1 handful fresh parsley

Place all the ingredients into the feed tube of your juicer. Juice according to the manufacturer's directions. Pour the fresh juice into a glass and enjoy immediately.

Yield: about 2 cups

VERY BERRY CHIA SMOOTHIE

Phase 1 *Detox*

Low FODMAP

Enjoy this smoothie during all phases of the Elimination Diet—it's rich in powerful antioxidant compounds called anthocyanins! When you are entering phase 3 and challenging oranges and citrus, add one whole peeled orange to this smoothie.

1 cup frozen wild blueberries	2 to 3 cups water
1 cup frozen cranberries	2 tablespoons chia seeds
1 cup frozen strawberries	1 small bunch black kale

Place all the ingredients in a high-powered blender and blend until smooth and creamy. Store any leftover smoothie in a glass jar in the refrigerator for up to 2 days.

Yield: about 6 cups

GINGER-BERRY SMOOTHIE

Phase 3 *Reintroduction (oranges)*

Low FODMAP

Use this smoothie recipe when challenging citrus in phase 3. This smoothie, or a variation of it, is what we make most often at home for breakfast or snacks. Sometimes we will use tangerines or mandarins in place of the oranges. If there are a lot of seeds in the oranges, you can easily get them out by slicing the oranges in half after they have been peeled, and then using the tip of a knife to pop them out.

3 cups water

½ to 1 bunch collard greens

2½ cups fresh or frozen blueberries

1 cup fresh or frozen pitted cherries

2 small oranges, peeled

1 (2-inch) piece fresh ginger

Place all the ingredients in a high-powered blender and blend until smooth. Serve immediately. Store any leftover smoothie in a glass jar in the refrigerator for up to 2 days.

Yield: about 7 cups

RED CABBAGE AND BERRY SMOOTHIE

Phase 1 *Detox*

I like adding chia seeds and avocado to smoothies to add more fat and calories, which helps to maintain satiety. This antioxidant-packed smoothie has a beautiful purplish-red color and is full of berry flavors. Be sure not to add more than 3 cups coarsely chopped cabbage; otherwise, the flavor gets too strong!

¼ head small red cabbage (2 to 3 cups chopped)

1 small avocado

2 cups fresh or frozen blueberries

2 cups fresh or frozen pitted cherries

1 cup fresh or frozen raspberries

½ cup fresh or frozen cranberries

2 tablespoons chia seeds

3 cups water

Place all the ingredients in a high-powered blender and blend until smooth and creamy. Add more water for a thinner smoothie. Serve immediately.

Yield: about 8 cups

STRAWBERRY-KALE-MINT SMOOTHIE

Phase 1 *Detox*

Low FODMAP

We love harvesting strawberries from local organic farms in the summertime and then freezing them to use throughout the year. Try this summertime smoothie using either fresh or frozen fruit. Sometimes I will add in half of an avocado or 2 tablespoons of chia seeds for extra healthy fats.

2 cups fresh or frozen strawberries	½ to 1 bunch black kale
2 cups chopped pineapple	1 small handful fresh mint
2 cups water	1 to 2 tablespoons chia seeds

Place all the ingredients in a high-powered blender and blend until smooth. Taste and add more kale, if desired; blend again. Drink immediately.

Yield: about 6 cups

Phase 3 VARIATION

To use this to test citrus in phase 3, add the juice of 1 lime to this recipe.

PINEAPPLE GREEN SMOOTHIE

Phase 1 *Detox*

This is another fantastic smoothie to enjoy during all phases of the diet—it's one of our favorites!

½ fresh pineapple, peeled and chopped (about 3 cups)	1 small handful fresh mint
	1 large handful fresh cilantro (optional)
1 small avocado, pitted and peeled	
½ bunch kale	2 to 3 cups coconut water or water

Place all the ingredients in a high-powered blender and blend until smooth. Taste and add more pineapple or kale, if desired; blend again. Drink immediately.

Yield: about 6 cups

Phase 3 VARIATION
To test citrus in phase 3, add the juice of 1 lime to this recipe.

BERRY VANILLA MILKSHAKE

Phase 3 *Reintroduction (nuts)*

Use this smoothie when challenging nuts in phase 3. If you've found you don't do well with cashews, replace them with an equal amount of raw almonds that have been soaked for 8 hours in filtered water. This nutrient-dense smoothie keeps me going strong for hours without feeling hungry! If you would like it a little sweeter, add half of a banana or two pitted Medjool dates.

½ cup raw cashews	½ teaspoon raw vanilla powder
¼ cup raw Brazil nuts	2 cups water
2 tablespoons hemp seeds	1 cup frozen blueberries
1 tablespoon chia seeds	1 cup frozen pitted cherries

Place all the ingredients except for the blueberries and cherries in a high-powered blender and blend until smooth and creamy. Add the blueberries and cherries and blend again until smooth. Serve immediately.

Yield: 4 cups

STRAWBERRY-ALMOND MILKSHAKE

Phase 3 *Reintroduction (almonds)*

Use this tasty dairy-free milkshake recipe when challenging almonds in phase 3. Soaking almonds overnight makes them far more digestible and unlocks many of their nutrients. This is what happens when you plant a seed in the earth and then water it—it wakes up and prepares to germinate, unlocking its nutrients for use in growing into a plant. Serve this smoothie as a snack or as a light breakfast.

½ cup raw almonds

2 cups filtered water

1 small frozen banana

2 cups fresh or frozen strawberries

¼ teaspoon raw vanilla powder (optional)

Place the almonds in a small bowl and cover them with filtered water. Let them soak on your counter overnight or for 8 to 10 hours. Then drain and rinse the almonds, and place them in a high-powered blender along with the 2 cups water. Blend on high until smooth and creamy. Add the banana, strawberries, and vanilla, if desired, and blend again until smooth. Serve immediately.

Yield: about 4½ cups

TIP

We buy glass and stainless steel smoothie straws and keep them handy for smoothies like this one—much better for the environment than plastic!

CHOCOLATE-AVOCADO MILKSHAKE

Phase 3 *Reintroduction (nuts, chocolate)*

Use this recipe during phase 3 after you have introduced nuts and are challenging chocolate. It's a nutrient-dense, energizing smoothie that works well for breakfast or as an afternoon snack. I like to add a little bit of raw manuka honey to smoothies because of its amazing ability to boost the immune system. You can omit it or use regular raw honey instead. Brazil nuts are a very rich source of selenium, a mineral needed for proper detoxification and immune system function.

½ cup raw Brazil nuts

2 cups water

2 small frozen bananas

½ avocado

2 to 4 Medjool dates, pitted

¼ cup raw cacao powder

1 tablespoon chia seeds

1 tablespoon raw manuka honey or other raw honey

½ teaspoon raw vanilla powder

½ teaspoon ground cinnamon

pinch sea salt

Place the Brazil nuts and water in a high-powered blender and blend until smooth. Add the remaining ingredients, then blend until supersmooth. Drink immediately or pour into Popsicle molds and freeze to have as a treat later.

Yield: about 4 cups

BREAKFAST

CREAMY RICE CEREAL

Phase 2 *Elimination*

Low FODMAP

This is one of our children's favorite breakfasts, and it's in high demand in our house. We use whole, organic, sprouted brown rice and then grind it in the dry container of our Vitamix. You can also use a coffee grinder (one that's not used for coffee) to grind the rice into a fine meal. Serve with a sprinkling of coconut sugar, ground cinnamon, and frozen blueberries.

1 cup uncooked brown rice pinch sea salt
4 cups water

Grind the brown rice in a high-powered blender or coffee grinder to a fine meal. It should be a little coarser than rice flour. Transfer it to a small pot along with the water and sea salt; whisk together well and set over high heat. Bring to a boil, whisking continuously then reduce the heat to low, cover, and simmer, whisking occasionally, for 10 to 15 minutes. Serve.

Yield: 3 to 4 servings

COCONUT-QUINOA BREAKFAST PORRIDGE

Phase 2 *Elimination*

Low FODMAP

This quinoa porridge recipe is a rich and nutritious way to start your day. When you are challenging nuts in phase 3, you can adapt this recipe by replacing the coconut milk with homemade Raw Vanilla Almond Milk (page 290) or Vanilla Cashew Milk (page 291). When you are challenging dairy, replace the coconut milk with raw whole milk or cream.

1½ cups uncooked quinoa, rinsed and drained	**OPTIONAL TOPPINGS**
4 cups water	pure maple syrup or raw honey
1 cup coconut milk	coconut sugar
¼ teaspoon sea salt	hemp seeds
1 cup fresh or frozen blueberries	chia seeds
	cinnamon

Place the quinoa, water, coconut milk, and sea salt in a 2-quart pot, cover, and bring to a gentle boil. Reduce the heat to a simmer and cook for about 20 minutes. Stir in the blueberries and cook for 3 to 4 minutes more. Stir and serve hot with optional toppings of your choosing.

Yield: 6 servings

TURKEY, KALE, AND CARROT HASH

`Phase 2` *Elimination*

`Low FODMAP`

This breakfast will nourish and sustain you for hours! Make up a big batch on the weekend and then reheat small portions as needed in a small skillet with a few tablespoons of water. Serve over Baked Winter Squash (page 243) with a few spoonfuls of Rainbow Kraut (page 299). I also like to add sliced avocados to my portion or drizzle the whole meal with the Green Goddess Dressing (page 273).

1 tablespoon extra-virgin olive oil	3 to 4 green onions, cut into thin rounds
1 pound organic ground turkey	2 large carrots, grated
½ to 1 teaspoon sea salt	3 cups thinly sliced kale
½ teaspoon ground cumin	
½ teaspoon dried oregano	

Heat the oil in a deep 11- to 12-inch skillet over medium heat. Add the turkey, salt, cumin, and oregano; sauté for 3 to 5 minutes. Then add the green onions, carrots, and kale; continue to sauté until the vegetables are tender, 5 to 7 minutes more.

Taste and adjust the salt and seasonings if necessary.

Yield: 4 to 6 servings

TIP

This meal is especially beneficial for those experiencing starch maldigestion, FODMAP sensitivity, or SIBO.

Phase 3 VARIATION

Replace the ground turkey with an equal amount of organic grass-fed beef when challenging beef in phase 3.

SWEET POTATO–KALE HASH

Phase 2 *Elimination*

Try making a large batch of this on the weekend and then reheating small portions for breakfast throughout the week. Add leftover cooked salmon, chicken, turkey, or cooked beans for more protein.

2 tablespoons coconut oil or extra-virgin olive oil

4 cups diced sweet potatoes (about 2 medium)

1 teaspoon crushed dried sage

¼ teaspoon ground cumin

¼ teaspoon sea salt or Herbamare

freshly ground black pepper

3 to 4 cups chopped kale

4 to 5 green onions, sliced into rounds

Heat the oil in a 12-inch skillet over medium heat. Add the sweet potatoes, sage, cumin, salt, and pepper and sauté for 7 to 10 minutes, reducing the heat if necessary to prevent burning. Then add the kale and green onions and sauté for a few minutes more.

Test to see if the sweet potatoes are cooked through; if not, add a few tablespoons of water, put a lid on the pan, and continue to cook for a few more minutes until done.

Taste and adjust the salt and seasonings if necessary.

Yield: 4 to 6 servings

Phase 3 **VARIATION**

Add in 1 diced medium red bell pepper to the hash when challenging nightshades in phase 3.

LAMB-QUINOA BREAKFAST HASH

Phase 2 *Elimination*

This meal gives you sustained energy to last all morning long. Substitute ground turkey or cooked adzuki beans for the lamb, if desired. Serve with fresh organic salad greens or a fermented vegetable, such as the Pickled Cauliflower, Carrots, and Green Beans (page 297).

1 to 2 tablespoons extra-virgin olive oil	½ teaspoon freshly ground black pepper
1 small onion, diced	1 pound ground lamb
2 medium zucchini, diced	2 cups cooked quinoa
2 teaspoons dried Italian herbs	1 cup chopped fresh parsley
1 teaspoon sea salt or Herbamare	

Heat the oil in a 12-inch cast-iron skillet over medium-low heat. Add the onion and sauté for about 10 minutes, or until golden. Add the zucchini and sauté for about 5 minutes more. Then add the dried herbs, salt or Herbamare, pepper, and lamb. Cook for 5 minutes more, or until the lamb is cooked through. Then add the quinoa and stir together. Turn off the heat and stir in the parsley. Taste and adjust the salt and seasonings, if desired.

Yield: about 6 servings

CHICKEN-APPLE BREAKFAST SAUSAGES

Phase 2 *Elimination*

You can make this recipe ahead of time, form the sausages into patties, and either freeze or refrigerate them before cooking. Then take one or two out at a time to cook as needed. Uncooked sausages will last for up to 2 days in the refrigerator or 6 months in the freezer. Serve with a green salad and a cup of herbal tea for breakfast. You can also serve these for dinner sandwiched between two romaine lettuce leaves with your favorite fixings!

1 medium tart apple, cored, peeled, and chopped	½ teaspoon freshly ground black pepper
5 green onions, cut into 1-inch pieces	1½ pounds organic skinless, boneless chicken thighs
3 tablespoons fresh sage leaves	
1 teaspoon Herbamare or sea salt	extra-virgin olive oil or coconut oil, for cooking

Place the apple, green onions, sage, salt, and pepper in a food processor fitted with the "s" blade and pulse a few times. Then add the chicken and process until the chicken is ground and the mixture starts to form a ball. It does not take long, only about 30 seconds.

With oiled hands, form the mixture into about 8 patties and set them on a plate or baking sheet. Heat a large cast-iron skillet over medium-low heat, then add about 1 tablespoon oil. Place four of the patties in the pan and cook for 4 to 5 minutes on each side. Repeat with the remaining patties. Serve.

Yield: 8 sausage patties

KALE, ZUCCHINI, AND EGG SCRAMBLE

Phase 3 *Reintroduction (eggs)*

Low FODMAP

Use this recipe for challenging eggs in phase 3. Be sure to use either organic or pastured eggs during the three-day egg challenge! This simple recipe takes just minutes to prepare and will leave you feeling energized all morning long. Serve with a spoonful of raw cultured vegetables to maximize digestion.

2 teaspoons coconut oil, plus more as needed

1 medium zucchini, diced

2 cups finely chopped kale

4 large organic eggs

sea salt and freshly ground black pepper

2 tablespoons minced fresh parsley

Heat a 10-inch skillet over medium heat. Add the coconut oil. Then add the diced zucchini and chopped kale. Sauté for about 5 minutes, adding a tablespoon or two of water if needed to help the kale soften.

While the veggies are cooking, crack the eggs into a bowl and whisk. Before adding the eggs, push the zucchini and kale to the side of the pan and add a few more teaspoons of coconut oil. This will prevent the eggs from sticking to the bottom of the pan while cooking. Add the eggs and scramble them into the veggies. Cook, turning constantly, for about 2 minutes.

Remove from the heat and season with salt and pepper to taste. Garnish with the parsley.

Yield: 2 to 4 servings

CELERIAC-RUTABAGA HASH BROWNS

Phase 2 *Elimination*

Low FODMAP

Other root vegetables can replace potatoes when making hash browns. My favorite is to use a combination of celeriac and rutabaga. I cut the vegetables into pieces and then use my food processor fitted with the grating disc to quickly grate everything. You should have 4 to 5 cups total. Serve with Chicken-Apple Breakfast Sausages (page 202) and organic salad greens for a balanced meal.

¼ cup extra-virgin olive oil or coconut oil	1 medium celeriac, peeled and grated
sea salt and freshly ground black pepper	1 medium rutabaga, peeled and grated

Heat a 10-inch cast-iron skillet over medium-low heat. Once it's hot, add the oil and sprinkle the bottom of the pan with salt and pepper. Then add the grated vegetables. Cook for 10 to 20 minutes without stirring. You want to make sure that the heat is low enough so the vegetables don't burn but hot enough so they cook properly. Adjust accordingly.

Flip the hash browns using a large, wide spatula and cook for 10 to 15 minutes more. Taste and add more salt and pepper, if necessary. Serve.

Yield: about 4 servings

SPICED SEED GRANOLA

Phase 2 *Elimination*

Low FODMAP

Carry a small container of this grain-free seed-based granola with you for a snack or serve it for breakfast with Vanilla Hemp Milk (page 290) topped with fresh berries. When shopping for seeds, look for shelled green pumpkin seeds, often called pepitas.

2 cups raw pumpkin seeds	¼ teaspoon sea salt
2 cups raw sunflower seeds	¼ cup pure maple syrup
3 tablespoons chia seeds	¼ cup melted coconut oil
2 teaspoons ground cinnamon	½ to 1 cup dried currants (optional)
½ to 1 teaspoon ground ginger	

Preheat the oven to 300°F. Line a large, rimmed baking sheet with parchment paper.

Place the pumpkin seeds and sunflower seeds in a food processor fitted with the "s" blade. Process until you have a chunky, coarse meal. Pour into a medium mixing bowl and add the chia seeds, cinnamon, ginger, and salt; stir together. Then add the maple syrup and coconut oil; stir together well.

Spread the mixture out onto the prepared baking sheet and bake for about 35 minutes, turning the granola over about halfway through baking. Remove from the oven and stir in the currants, if using. Let cool completely to crisp up. Then transfer to a glass jar and store on your counter for up to 10 days.

Yield: about 4 cups

CREAMY GREEN DETOX SOUP

Phase 1 *Detox*

Use this soup during the first two days of detoxing and throughout the entire diet—it's easy to digest, light, and nourishing. Add additional fresh herbs, if desired—try dill, tarragon, or oregano. Freeze cooled soup (see page 102) in widemouthed pint or quart jars for later use.

1 tablespoon extra-virgin olive oil	2 to 3 teaspoons Herbamare or sea salt
1 large leek, chopped	
2 pounds zucchini, chopped	2 teaspoons dried thyme
1 pound green beans, trimmed	1 bunch fresh spinach (about 4 cups packed), rinsed
6 to 8 cups water, Chicken Stock (page 295), or Vegetable-Seaweed Stock (page 296)	
	1 large handful fresh parsley
	1 large handful fresh basil

Heat the oil in a 6- to 8-quart pot over medium heat. Add the leek and sauté for about 5 minutes. Then add the zucchini, green beans, water, Herbamare, and thyme. Cover and simmer for about 15 minutes, or until the vegetables are tender. Add the spinach, parsley, and basil; cover and simmer for 2 minutes more. Then remove the pot from the heat and use an immersion blender to purée the soup right in the pot, or carefully transfer the soup to a blender and purée in batches.

Yield: about 8 servings

TIP

To chop a leek, first trim off the roots at the bottom, and then trim off the upper 1 to 2 inches. Slice the leek lengthwise down the center. Run it under cold water to remove the dirt, and then chop.

CARROT-GINGER-SHIITAKE SOUP

Phase 1 *Detox*

We prefer to use quite a bit more ginger in this soup than what I call for here. If you love the flavor and spice that ginger provides, then add up to a 4-inch piece of ginger. If your ginger is quite fresh, there is no need to peel it; if it is older with a thick skin, then peel it. Enjoy this soup during all phases of the Elimination Diet.

1 to 2 tablespoons extra-virgin olive oil

1 small onion, diced

1 (2-inch) piece fresh ginger, chopped

10 shiitake mushrooms, chopped

2 pounds carrots, peeled and chopped

6 cups Chicken Stock (page 295) or Vegetable-Seaweed Stock (page 296)

2 teaspoons Herbamare or sea salt

GARNISHES

sautéed shiitake mushroom slices

chopped fresh cilantro

Heat the oil in a 6-quart pot over medium heat. Add the onions and sauté until soft, about 7 minutes. Then add the remaining ingredients except for the garnishes, cover, and simmer for about 30 minutes.

Use an immersion blender to purée the soup in the pot, or carefully transfer the soup to a blender and purée in batches. Top each bowl of soup with sautéed shiitake mushrooms and chopped cilantro.

Yield: about 6 servings

BEET-ROSEMARY DETOX SOUP

Phase 1 *Detox*

Use this soup during all phases of the diet—it's nourishing, warming, and full of compounds that assist the liver in detoxification.

2 tablespoons extra-virgin olive oil	2 to 3 tablespoons chopped fresh rosemary
1 medium onion, chopped	
4 garlic cloves, peeled and chopped	1 handful fresh parsley
2 to 3 medium beets, peeled and chopped	2 teaspoons sea salt or Herbamare
	6 cups water or Vegetable-Seaweed Stock (page 296)
5 large carrots, peeled and chopped	
	chopped fresh parsley, for garnish (optional)

Heat the oil in a 6-quart pot over medium heat. Add the onion and sauté for 5 to 10 minutes, until soft and beginning to change color. Add the remaining ingredients except for the parsley, cover, and simmer for about 30 minutes.

Purée the soup in the pot using an immersion blender, or carefully transfer the soup to a blender and purée in batches until smooth and creamy. Taste and adjust the salt and seasonings if necessary. Garnish with chopped fresh parsley, if desired.

Yield: about 6 servings

Phase 3 **VARIATION**

When you enter the last stages of the diet, top each bowl of soup with a dollop of organic sour cream as part of the dairy challenge.

CREAMY BROCCOLI-MUSHROOM SOUP

Phase 1 *Detox*

Use this soup during all phases of the diet; it is simple to make and easy to digest. Try adding other vegetables, such as zucchini, garlic, parsnips, kale, or spinach. Add extra stock if you add extra vegetables.

1 to 2 tablespoons extra-virgin olive oil

1 large leek, chopped

1½ pounds broccoli, chopped

8 ounces cremini mushrooms, chopped

6 cups Chicken Stock (page 295) or Vegetable-Seaweed Stock (page 296)

2 teaspoons dried thyme

1 tablespoon fresh oregano leaves

1 handful fresh parsley

1 handful fresh basil

sea salt and freshly ground black pepper

Heat the oil in a 6-quart pot over medium heat. Add the leek and sauté for about 5 minutes, or until softened. Then add the broccoli, mushrooms, stock, and thyme. Cover and simmer for about 20 minutes, or until the vegetables are tender.

Turn off the heat and add the fresh herbs. Purée the soup in the pot using an immersion blender, or carefully transfer the soup to a blender and purée in batches. Season with salt and pepper to taste. Serve. Freeze soup in wide-mouthed quart or pint jars (see page 102), if desired.

Yield: about 6 servings

CREAMY CAULIFLOWER-PARSNIP SOUP

Phase 1 *Detox*

If parsnips are out of season, use extra cauliflower, or try zucchini, carrots, or broccoli. Use a homemade chicken or turkey stock for best results.

2 tablespoons extra-virgin olive oil

1 large leek, chopped

2 to 3 parsnips, peeled and chopped

1 large head cauliflower (about 2 pounds), chopped

8 cups Chicken Stock (page 295) or Vegetable-Seaweed Stock (page 296)

2 teaspoons dried thyme

2 teaspoons Herbamare or sea salt

¼ teaspoon freshly ground black pepper

½ cup chopped fresh parsley

Heat the oil in a 6- to 8-quart pot over medium heat. Add the leek and sauté until softened, about 5 minutes. Then add the parsnips, cauliflower, stock, thyme, Herbamare, and pepper. Cover the pot, bring to a boil over medium heat, then reduce the heat to low and simmer for about 20 minutes.

Remove the pot from the heat. Purée the soup in the pot using an immersion blender, or carefully transfer the soup to a blender and purée in batches. Stir in the parsley. Serve.

Yield: 6 to 8 servings

ADZUKI BEAN AND SEA VEGETABLE SOUP

Phase 2 *Elimination*

Serve this nourishing soup for breakfast, lunch, or dinner. You can make this on the stovetop or in your slow cooker. Although adzuki beans don't need to be soaked before cooking, I have found that when using the slow cooker, you need to soak them first in order for them to cook properly. Before you go to work or school in the morning, place your beans in a bowl and cover with filtered water. Then before you go to bed that night, drain the beans and place them in your slow cooker with the rest of the ingredients. You will wake up to a pot of warm soup to serve for breakfast or pack for lunch! Serve this soup with a dollop of sticky brown rice, if desired.

1 tablespoon extra-virgin olive oil

1 small onion, diced

1½ cups adzuki beans (soaked for 8 to 12 hours)

3 to 4 garlic cloves, crushed

1 (1-inch) piece fresh ginger, grated

3 carrots, diced

2 celery stalks, diced

8 to 10 shiitake mushrooms, sliced

1 to 2 strips wakame seaweed, broken into small pieces

8 cups Chicken Stock (page 295) or Vegetable-Seaweed Stock (page 296)

2 teaspoons sea salt

OPTIONAL GARNISHES

chopped fresh cilantro

raw coconut vinegar

coconut aminos

soy-free, gluten-free miso

If you are making this recipe on the stovetop, heat the oil in a 6-quart pot over medium heat. Add the onion and sauté for about 5 minutes, or until softened. Add the remaining ingredients except for the garnishes, cover, and simmer for about 45 minutes.

If you are using a slow cooker, heat the oil in a 10-inch skillet over medium heat. Add the onion and sauté for about 5 minutes, or until softened. Transfer the sautéed onion to the slow cooker and then add the remaining ingredients except for the garnishes, cover, and cook on low for 8 hours or high for 4 to 5 hours.

To test and see if the beans are cooked, you can take a few out and mash them between your fingers. They should be soft and mash easily. If not, continue to cook until done. Serve with optional garnishes.

Yield: 6 to 8 servings

TIP

Did you know that sea vegetables offer a concentrated source of trace minerals, particularly iodine? Iodine is needed to make thyroid hormone. Thyroid hormone is incredibly important for normal function of the human body. So important that every single cell has a receptor for this amazing "master switch" of metabolism. Want to have perfectly regulated body weight and body temperature? Then shoot for optimal thyroid hormone function. How do you do that? Eat a gluten-free, whole-foods diet that keeps your autoimmune thyroid antibodies down, and include seaweed in your diet on an occasional basis.

MUNG BEAN, ZUCCHINI, AND DILL SOUP

Phase 3 *Reintroduction (citrus)*

Serve this flavorful, nourishing soup with a scoop of cooked quinoa or brown rice and a large green salad. This recipe contains lemon juice. Use it to challenge citrus in phase 3 or omit the lemon and use this recipe during phase 2.

1 to 2 tablespoons extra-virgin olive oil	1 teaspoon kelp granules (optional)
1 small onion, diced	2 medium zucchini, diced
1½ cups dry mung beans	3 to 4 cups chopped fresh spinach
10 cups water or Vegetable-Seaweed Stock (page 296)	½ cup chopped fresh dill
1 to 2 teaspoons dried thyme	2 teaspoons Herbamare or sea salt
	juice of 1 lemon (optional)

Heat the oil in a 4- to 6-quart pot over medium heat. Add the onion and sauté for about 5 minutes. Then add the mung beans, water, thyme, and kelp granules, if using. Cover the pot and simmer for about 30 minutes.

Add the zucchini and simmer for 5 to 7 minutes more. Add the spinach, dill, salt, and lemon, if using. Simmer for a few minutes more. Taste and adjust the salt and seasonings, if desired.

Yield: 6 to 8 servings

WHITE BEAN, WILD RICE, AND KALE SOUP

Phase 2 *Elimination*

This hearty, warming soup is perfect to make on a chilly autumn or winter evening. We like to use cannellini beans, but other white beans, such as navy or great northern, work as well. Serve with the Roasted Delicata Squash Salad with Apples and Toasted Pumpkin Seeds (page 231) for a balanced meal. This soup freezes well—see page 102 for instructions for freezing soup.

12 cups Vegetable-Seaweed Stock (page 296) or Chicken Stock (page 295)	4 cups chopped kale
	½ cup chopped fresh parsley
1 cup uncooked wild rice	1 to 2 tablespoons chopped fresh rosemary
1 medium onion, diced	
3 large carrots, diced	2 to 3 teaspoons sea salt or Herbamare
4 celery stalks, chopped	
3 cups cooked white beans	½ teaspoon freshly ground black pepper

In an 8-quart pot, bring the stock to a gentle boil. Add the rice and onion, cover, and simmer for about 40 minutes. Then add the carrots, celery, and white beans; simmer for 15 to 20 minutes more.

Add the kale, parsley, rosemary, salt, and pepper; simmer for about 5 minutes more. Taste and adjust the salt and seasonings, if desired.

Yield: 8 to 10 servings

VARIATION

Replace the white beans with chopped cooked chicken.

SIMPLE VEGETABLE SOUP

`Phase 2` *Elimination*

This soup makes the perfect breakfast on day 3 when you are coming off of phase 1. Keep a few jars in your fridge at all times to have on hand for quick meals on the go. Feel free to use 8 cups of your favorite vegetables—try the combination I suggest below or your own creation!

1 tablespoon extra-virgin olive oil
1 cup chopped leeks
1 cup diced onions
8 cups chopped mixed vegetables (carrots, celery, mushrooms, zucchini)
6 cups Chicken Stock (page 295)
3 cups chopped kale
½ cup chopped fresh parsley

sea salt and freshly ground black pepper

OPTIONAL ADDITIONS
sautéed ground organic chicken or turkey
shredded cooked organic chicken or turkey breast
1 tablespoon dried hijiki or arame
1 tablespoon grated fresh ginger

Heat the oil in a 4- to 6-quart pot over medium heat. Add the leeks and onion; sauté for 3 to 5 minutes. Add the mixed vegetables and stock, as well as any optional additions; cover and simmer for 10 to 15 minutes, or until vegetables are tender. Add the kale and parsley; simmer for 4 to 5 minutes more. Season with salt and pepper to taste.

Yield: 4 to 6 servings

HEALING CABBAGE AND CHICKEN SOUP

Phase 2 *Elimination*

Once you have made a few large batches of both the Chicken Stock (page 295) and the Vegetable-Seaweed Stock (page 296), anything is possible when it comes to soup. Using one of those stocks as a base, you can quickly whip up a pot of soup that can nourish you throughout the week. This recipe can be made very quickly; serve it with leftover cooked brown or white jasmine rice.

6 cups Vegetable-Seaweed Stock (page 296) or Chicken Stock (page 295)

¾ pound organic skinless, boneless chicken thighs, cut into thin strips

2 teaspoons grated fresh ginger

1 to 2 teaspoons sea salt

1 small daikon radish, peeled and sliced into thin rounds

2 large carrots, peeled and sliced into thin rounds

4 cups chopped napa cabbage

GARNISHES

½ cup chopped fresh cilantro

3 to 4 green onions, cut into thin rounds

crushed red chili flakes (add only when challenging nightshades in phase 3 or if you can tolerate nightshades)

In a 4-quart pot, bring the stock to a gentle boil. Add the chicken, ginger, salt, daikon radish, and carrots, cover, reduce the heat to low, and simmer for 15 to 20 minutes. Add the napa cabbage and simmer for a few minutes more. Taste and adjust the salt, if desired. Ladle the soup into bowls and sprinkle each with the garnishes as desired.

Yield: 6 servings

Phase 3 **VARIATION**

Replace the chicken with cubed organic tofu when you are challenging soy at the end of phase 3.

SUMMER VEGETABLE SOUP

Phase 3 *Reintroduction (nightshades)*

Make this soup when challenging tomatoes and other nightshade vegetables during phase 3. It's just perfect for a chilly summer evening.

2 tablespoons extra-virgin olive oil

1 medium sweet onion, diced

4 medium zucchini or pattypan squash, diced

2 cups chopped green beans

2 large tomatoes, diced

1 bunch kale, chopped (4 to 5 cups)

1 to 2 teaspoons dried tarragon

1 to 2 teaspoons dried thyme

10 cups Chicken Stock (page 295) or Vegetable-Seaweed Stock (page 296)

1 large handful fresh parsley, chopped

2 to 3 teaspoons sea salt or Herbamare

freshly ground black pepper

OPTIONAL ADDITIONS

2 cups cooked chickpeas

2 cups cooked red beans

2 cups cooked quinoa

2 cups chopped cooked chicken breast

Heat the oil in an 8-quart pot over medium heat. Add the onion; sauté for 5 to 7 minutes, or until softened. Add the zucchini, green beans, tomatoes, kale, tarragon, thyme, and stock. Stir, cover, and bring to a boil. Once boiling, immediately reduce the heat to low and simmer for about 15 minutes, or until the vegetables are tender.

Add the parsley, salt, and pepper, as well as any optional additions; simmer for 3 to 4 minutes more. Remove the pot from the heat, taste, and adjust the salt and herbs, if necessary. Serve.

Yield: 6 to 8 servings

TIP

1 teaspoon dried herbs equals 1 tablespoon of fresh herbs. Replace the dried herbs in this recipe with 1 to 2 tablespoons of chopped fresh!

CHICKEN VEGETABLE SOUP

Phase 2 *Elimination*

Make a pot of this soup on the weekend so you will have ready-to-go food during the week. You can vary this recipe by adding different vegetables to the soup portion. Try shiitake mushrooms, lemongrass, and grated ginger for an Asian-inspired soup. You could also add diced root vegetables such as parsnips, rutabagas, celeriac, turnips, and golden beets for a winter vegetable chicken soup.

BROTH

1 (3- to 4-pound) whole organic chicken

1 onion, chopped

1 head garlic, cut in half crosswise

3 celery stalks, chopped

1 carrot, chopped

3 to 4 sprigs fresh thyme

2 sprigs fresh rosemary

1 to 2 teaspoons whole black peppercorns

1 bay leaf

1 tablespoon sea salt

12 cups filtered water

SOUP

1 small onion, diced

1 small leek, chopped

3 to 4 large carrots, diced

3 to 4 celery stalks, diced

½ pound green beans, trimmed and cut into 2-inch pieces

2 to 3 teaspoons dried thyme

3 to 4 cups chopped kale

½ cup chopped fresh parsley

sea salt and freshly ground black pepper

To make the broth, place the chicken in an 8-quart pot. Add the remaining ingredients for the broth. Cover and simmer for 1 to 2 hours on low heat. Place a colander over another large pot. Pour the broth through the colander. Let it drain well. Then place the broth back on the stove. Carefully remove the whole chicken (it will be hot) from the colander and place it on a plate to cool. Discard the other solids.

To make the soup, place the onion, leek, carrots, celery, green beans, and thyme into the pot with the broth. Cover and simmer for 15 to 20 minutes, or until the vegetables are tender.

Pull all of the meat from the bones of the chicken and cut larger pieces into smaller ones. Add the chicken meat to the pot with the simmering vegetables. Then add the kale and parsley and simmer for about 5 minutes more. Season with salt and ground black pepper as desired. Serve.

Yield: 10 to 12 servings

VARIATION

Add 1 package partially cooked quinoa-rice spaghetti noodles to this soup when you add the chicken back to the soup.

TURKEY VEGETABLE SOUP

Phase 2 *Elimination*

This soup makes for a warming winter meal. Add 3 to 4 cups cooked wild rice for a heartier soup, if desired. Making soup with bone-in, skin-on poultry is a two-part process—first, you make a rich broth, then you make the soup. It's very simple, but it does require a few hours of cooking time, so plan on making this soup on the weekend.

BROTH
10 to 12 cups water
1 (2½ to 3-pound) organic bone-in, skin-on turkey breast
1 small onion, chopped
1 head garlic, cut in half crosswise
1 large carrot, chopped
2 to 3 celery stalks, chopped
2 to 3 sprigs fresh rosemary
2 bay leaves
1 tablespoon sea salt
1 teaspoon whole black peppercorns

SOUP
1 small onion or leek, chopped
2 cups diced carrots
2 cups diced celery
2 cups chopped green beans
3 to 4 cups diced butternut squash
2 teaspoons dried thyme
1 teaspoon crushed dried sage
4 cups baby spinach leaves
1 handful fresh parsley, chopped

To make the broth, place all the ingredients for the broth into an 8-quart pot and bring to a boil. Cover, reduce the heat to a low simmer, and cook for about 2 hours, or until the meat easily falls off the bone.

When the turkey is cooked, place a colander over a large clean pot and strain the broth through it. Transfer the turkey breast to a plate to cool. Discard the remaining solids in the colander. Set the pot of broth on the stovetop.

To make the soup, add the onion, carrots, celery, green beans, squash, thyme, and sage to the pot with the strained broth. Simmer over medium-low heat for 20 minutes, or until the vegetables are tender.

While the vegetables are simmering, remove the skin from the turkey and pull the meat from the bones. Cut the meat into pieces and then add it to the pot with the simmering vegetables.

Add the baby spinach and parsley; stir well. Remove the soup from the heat, taste, and adjust the salt or seasonings, if desired.

Yield: 10 to 12 servings

SWEET POTATO, FENNEL, AND CHICKEN STEW

Phase 2 *Elimination*

Serve this warming soup on a chilly autumn evening with a few spoonfuls of fermented vegetables or a large green salad for a balanced meal.

---

2 tablespoons extra-virgin olive oil

1 large onion, chopped

1 large fennel bulb, chopped

1 teaspoon Herbamare or sea salt

3 to 4 teaspoons dried thyme

1½ pounds organic skinless, boneless chicken thighs

8 cups Chicken Stock (page 295)

6 cups chopped, peeled sweet potatoes (about 3 small)

1 medium golden beet, peeled and diced

1 medium delicata squash, seeded and chopped

½ cup chopped fresh parsley

Heat the oil in an 8-quart pot over medium heat. Add the onion, fennel, and Herbamare; cook for 10 to 12 minutes, or until the vegetables are very soft. Then add the thyme, chicken, stock, and sweet potatoes; cover and simmer for about 40 minutes.

Use the back of a long-handled spoon to gently mash the sweet potatoes so they fall apart. Eventually they will completely cook down to make a beautiful, creamy soup base. Add the beet and delicata squash; cover and simmer for about 40 minutes more.

Add the parsley. Taste and adjust the salt and seasonings if necessary.

Yield: 6 to 8 servings

HARVEST SQUASH SOUP

Phase 2 *Elimination*

This soup makes a very quick meal as long as you have leftover cooked chicken and baked squash sitting in your refrigerator needing to be used up. I like to use the leftover meat from a whole roasted chicken. Use any type of winter squash—sugar pie pumpkins, butternut squash, Hubbard, acorn, or kabocha. The key to a flavorful soup is starting with a really rich homemade chicken or turkey stock! When you are entering phase 3 of the diet and challenging citrus, add a squeeze of lime to each bowl.

5 to 6 cups Chicken Stock (page 295)	5 green onions, sliced into thin rounds
2 to 3 cups mashed cooked winter squash	3 cups chopped kale, chard, or spinach
2 to 3 garlic cloves	2 teaspoons Herbamare or sea salt
1 teaspoon ground cumin	**GARNISH**
½ teaspoon ground cinnamon	chopped fresh cilantro
2 cups chopped cooked chicken	

Place the stock, squash, garlic, cumin, and cinnamon in a blender and purée until smooth. Transfer the soup to a 6-quart pot and bring to a gentle simmer over medium heat. Then add the chicken, green onions, kale, and salt; cover and simmer for about 10 minutes, or until the kale is tender. Taste and adjust the salt and seasonings if necessary. Garnish with cilantro.

Yield: 6 to 8 servings

Phase 3 **VARIATION**

Add lime wedges to garnish if challenging citrus in Phase 3.

Low FODMAP **VARIATION**

Use kabocha squash in this recipe—one of the only varieties of winter squash low in FODMAPs.

NIGHTSHADE-FREE BEEF STEW

Phase 3 *Reintroduction (beef)*

Use this recipe when reintroducing beef in phase 3. The pomegranate juice in this recipe is what I use to replace the acidity tomatoes usually give to beef stew. Look for pure, unsweetened pomegranate juice, not a blend of juices. Serve with baked winter squash and a large green salad for a balanced meal.

2 pounds grass-fed organic beef stew meat

1 small onion, chopped

3 to 4 carrots, cut into thick slices

3 to 4 celery stalks, cut into 2-inch pieces

2 medium rutabagas, peeled and cut into chunks

2 to 3 garlic cloves, crushed

1 teaspoon dried thyme

½ teaspoon crushed dried sage

½ teaspoon freshly ground black pepper

1½ to 2 teaspoons Herbamare

1 cup pure pomegranate juice

2 tablespoons arrowroot powder

½ cup chopped fresh parsley

Combine all the ingredients except the parsley in a 4-quart slow cooker. Cover and cook on high for 3 to 4 hours, or on low for 7 to 8 hours. Taste and adjust the salt and seasonings, if desired. Stir in the parsley. Serve.

Yield: about 6 servings

VARIATION

Replace the pomegranate juice with homemade beef stock.

QUINOA AND BLACK BEAN DOSAS

Phase 2 *Elimination*

Dosas are traditional Indian pancakes or crepes made from soaked and fermented whole grains and beans. They make a great bread replacement! Making dosas is a two-part process—first, you soak the grains and beans overnight, then you blend them into a batter and let it ferment. This is one of the most digestible ways to prepare grains and beans. Replace the black beans with adzuki beans, mung beans, black-eyed peas, or chickpeas.

DAY 1
1½ cups dry quinoa
¾ cup dry black beans
1 tablespoon apple cider vinegar
warm water to cover

DAY 2
1½ cups water
1 teaspoon sea salt

DAY 3 OR 4
virgin coconut oil for cooking

On day 1, rinse the quinoa in a fine-mesh strainer. Place it in a small mixing bowl along with the beans, apple cider vinegar, and warm water. Make sure there is at least an inch of water covering the quinoa and beans, as they will expand quite a bit during soaking. Let them soak for about 24 hours.

On day 2, drain and rinse the quinoa and beans and place them in a blender along with the water and salt; blend on high until smooth and creamy. Pour the mixture into a large clean mason jar or bowl, cover with a kitchen towel, and let the mixture ferment for 24 to 48 hours. It will turn slightly sour and a little bubbly.

When ready to cook, heat a cast-iron skillet over medium heat. Once it is hot, add a few teaspoons of coconut oil. Pour ⅓ to ½ cup of the batter into the hot skillet; spread it into a thin pancake in a circular motion using the back of a spoon. Cook for about 2 minutes on the first side, then flip and cook for about 1 minute on the other side. Place the dosa onto a plate. Continue with the remaining batter, adding coconut oil each time. Serve warm.

Yield: 8 to 10 dosas

BROWN RICE TORTILLAS

Phase 2 *Elimination*

This is one of the most popular recipes from our blog, NourishingMeals .com. Use these tortillas to make Black Bean, Yam, and Avocado Tacos (page 255) or Pomegranate Chicken Tacos (page 259). You can also serve them alongside your favorite soup or stew for dipping. They are soft and pliable when warm, but straight out of the fridge, like most gluten-free tortillas, they will crack. All you need to do to make them pliable again is to place one on a wire rack over a pot of simmering water and steam for 30 seconds on each side. I use an 8-inch cast-iron tortilla press to get them super thin, and then cook them in a cast-iron pan.

1¼ cups brown rice flour or sprouted brown rice flour	½ teaspoon sea salt
¾ cup arrowroot powder or tapioca flour	1 cup boiling water
	virgin coconut oil for cooking

In a small mixing bowl, whisk together the brown rice flour, arrowroot, and salt. Add the boiling water and quickly mix with a fork. Knead the dough a few times to form a ball. It should have the texture of Play-Doh. If it is too wet and sticky, add more flour. If it is too dry, add a little more boiling water.

Heat a 10-inch cast-iron skillet over medium heat. Divide the dough into six to eight equal-size balls. Place a piece of parchment paper on the bottom of a tortilla press, then place one of the balls in the center and cover with a second sheet of parchment. Press to form a thin, round tortilla.

Add about 1 teaspoon coconut oil to the hot skillet. Gently remove the parchment paper and place the tortilla in the hot skillet. Cook for 2 minutes on each side. Repeat with the remaining dough, adding more coconut oil to the skillet each time. Place the cooked tortillas on a plate with another plate flipped over on top of it to keep them warm and soft. Let them sit for about 20 minutes inside the plates; this way, they will be nice and pliable for serving.

Yield: 6 to 8 tortillas

ALMOND FLOUR TORTILLAS

Phase 3 *Reintroduction (almonds)*

Use this recipe for challenging almonds. These simple grain-free tortillas are very pliable and tasty! Serve them with your favorite fillings—chicken fajitas, beef tacos, hummus and grated vegetables, or whatever!

1 cup finely ground blanched almond flour

1 cup tapioca flour or arrowroot powder

½ teaspoon sea salt

½ cup boiling water

virgin coconut oil for cooking

In a small mixing bowl, whisk together the almond flour, tapioca, and salt. Add the boiling water and quickly mix with a fork. Knead the dough a few times to form a ball.

Heat a 10-inch cast-iron skillet over medium heat. Divide the dough into four to five equal-size balls. Place a piece of parchment paper on the bottom of a tortilla press, then place one of the balls in the center and cover with a second sheet of parchment. Press to form a thin, round tortilla.

Add about 1 teaspoon coconut oil to the hot skillet. Gently remove the parchment paper and place the tortilla in the hot skillet. Cook for 2 minutes on each side. Repeat with the remaining dough. Place the cooked tortillas on a plate with another plate flipped over on top of it to keep them warm and soft. Let them sit for about 10 minutes inside the plates; this way, they will be nice and pliable for serving.

Yield: 4 to 5 tortillas

BANANA MUFFINS

Phase 2 *Elimination*

These muffins are so simple to make and very satisfying. When you are challenging nuts in phase 3 or have tested okay for nuts, you can add ½ cup chopped walnuts to the batter. Try spreading a hot muffin with coconut butter and raw honey for a delicious sweet treat!

DRY INGREDIENTS

1½ cups brown rice flour or sprouted brown rice flour

¼ cup coconut sugar

1 teaspoon ground cinnamon

1 teaspoon baking soda

¼ teaspoon sea salt

WET INGREDIENTS

2 cups mashed ripe bananas (4 to 5 large)

½ cup melted coconut oil, plus more for greasing the dish

2 teaspoons raw apple cider vinegar

Preheat the oven to 350°F. Oil a 12-cup muffin pan with coconut oil or line it with unbleached paper liners.

Whisk together the dry ingredients in a medium mixing bowl. In a separate bowl, whisk together the wet ingredients. Pour the wet ingredients into the dry and vigorously mix together using a wooden spoon. Immediately fill each muffin cup about three quarters of the way full with the batter. Bake for 20 to 25 minutes. Cool on a wire rack.

Yield: 12 muffins

TIP

Use sprouted organic brown rice flour for the easiest digestibility and the most available nutrients.

CARROT BREAKFAST MUFFINS

Phase 3 *Reintroduction (almonds, eggs)*

Make this recipe after you have reintroduced and tested okay for almonds and are challenging eggs. Using high-protein almond flour and very little sweetener makes these muffins a good choice for breakfast. You will feel satiated longer because of the fat and protein found in the almond flour and eggs. Be sure to purchase "blanched almond flour," which is very finely ground.

DRY INGREDIENTS

2½ cups blanched almond flour
¾ teaspoon baking soda
¼ teaspoon sea salt
1 teaspoon ground cinnamon

WET INGREDIENTS

4 large organic eggs
1 medium ripe banana, mashed
  (¼ cup)
¼ cup melted coconut oil
2 tablespoons pure maple syrup or
  honey
1½ cups shredded carrots
¼ cup dried currants or raisins

Preheat the oven to 350°F. Line a 12-cup muffin pan with unbleached paper liners.

In a medium mixing bowl, whisk together the dry ingredients and set aside. In a smaller mixing bowl, whisk together the eggs, mashed banana, coconut oil, and maple syrup. Stir in the shredded carrots and currants. Pour the wet ingredients into the dry and mix together.

Scoop the batter by large spoonfuls into the prepared muffin pan. Bake for 30 to 35 minutes. Cool on a wire rack.

Yield: 12 muffins

SWEET POTATO SPICE MUFFINS

Phase 3 *Reintroduction (eggs)*

Use this recipe when reintroducing eggs in phase 3. Serve them for breakfast spread with coconut butter and honey along with sautéed kale and a Chicken-Apple Breakfast Sausage (page 202).

DRY INGREDIENTS
½ cup coconut flour
1 to 2 teaspoons ground cinnamon
½ teaspoon ground ginger
¾ teaspoon baking soda
¼ teaspoon sea salt

WET INGREDIENTS
5 large organic eggs
½ cup mashed cooked sweet potatoes
¼ cup melted coconut oil
¼ cup honey or pure maple syrup
1 teaspoon raw apple cider vinegar

Preheat the oven to 350°F. Line 9 wells of a 12-cup muffin pan with unbleached paper liners.

In a medium mixing bowl, whisk together the dry ingredients. In a separate mixing bowl, beat together the wet ingredients. Pour the wet ingredients into the dry and beat together.

Fill the prepared wells of the muffin pan about halfway with the batter. Bake for about 30 minutes. Cool on a wire rack. The muffins will last at room temperature in a covered container for about 4 days. Freeze for longer storage.

Yield: 9 muffins

CHIA-RICE SANDWICH BREAD

Phase 3 *Reintroduction (yeast)*

Low FODMAP

This delicious bread recipe is designed for the reintroduction of yeast during the late stages of phase 3. It's free of all other irritants, making it easy to notice if there is a reaction to yeast. If you find you are able to tolerate yeast, then use this bread recipe for sandwiches or toast (toasted in a dedicated gluten-free toaster) throughout the rest of the diet. Chia seeds can be found at most health food stores. Grind them in a coffee grinder or high-powered blender.

DRY INGREDIENTS

2½ to 3 cups brown rice flour or sprouted brown rice flour

1 cup arrowroot powder or tapioca flour

1¼ teaspoons sea salt

WET INGREDIENTS

2 cups warm water (105° to 110°F)

1 tablespoon pure maple syrup

1 tablespoon active dry yeast

½ cup ground chia seeds

Grease an 8.5 x 4.5-inch glass bread pan with coconut oil.

In a large mixing bowl, whisk together the dry ingredients. Set aside.

Place the water into a 4-cup glass liquid measuring cup or small glass mixing bowl. Add the maple syrup and yeast; whisk together. Let the yeast activate. It should get bubbly or foamy after about 5 minutes. Then vigorously whisk in the chia seeds.

Pour the wet ingredients into the dry and mix together with a wooden spoon. Continue to knead the dough with your hands until the ingredients are completely incorporated. It should feel a little moist and sticky. If it is so wet that it sticks to your hands, add more flour, a few tablespoons at a time, and knead until combined.

Place the dough into the bread pan and cover with a towel, plastic produce bag, or piece of waxed paper. Place the pan in a warm spot in your house and let the dough rise for about 1 hour.

Preheat the oven to 350°F. Bake the bread for about 50 minutes. Let cool in the pan for about 10 minutes, and then gently loosen the sides with a knife and transfer to a wire rack to cool.

Yield: 1 loaf

TIP

Use sprouted organic brown rice flour for the easiest digestibility and the most available nutrients.

GRATED RAW VEGETABLE BLISS SALAD

Phase 3 *Reintroduction (citrus)*

Prepare this salad during the beginning of phase 3 when challenging citrus. Use a food processor fitted with the grating disc to quickly grate all the vegetables. Serve this salad along with baked fish and cooked quinoa for a balanced meal.

SALAD

¼ head red cabbage, grated

¼ head green cabbage, grated

2 large carrots, grated

1 medium beet, grated

1 cup finely chopped fresh cilantro

3 to 4 green onions, sliced into thin rounds

DRESSING

¼ cup extra-virgin olive oil

finely grated zest of 1 lime

3 to 4 tablespoons freshly squeezed lime juice

2 to 3 teaspoons grated fresh ginger

1 to 2 garlic cloves, crushed

½ to 1 teaspoon Herbamare or sea salt

To make the salad, place all the ingredients for the salad into a large bowl.

To make the dressing, combine all the ingredients in a small jar, cover, and shake. Then pour the dressing over the salad, toss together, and serve.

Yield: about 8 servings

Phase 2 **VARIATION**

To make this salad acceptable for phase 2, simply omit the lime zest and replace the lime juice with either fermented vegetable brine or raw coconut vinegar.

SPRING SALAD WITH SNAP PEAS, SALMON, AND RADISHES

Phase 2 *Elimination*

I like to cook extra salmon when making dinner so I can have it to make big salads for lunch the next day. Use your favorite phase 2 salad dressing (see pages 271 to 276). I like to use the Green Goddess Dressing (page 273) with this salad.

---

8 cups organic mixed baby greens

1 to 2 cups cooked wild Alaskan salmon

1 bunch red radishes, cut into thin rounds

½ pound fresh sugar snap peas, chopped

2 to 3 green onions, sliced into thin rounds

½ cup chopped fresh parsley

Place the lettuce in a large salad bowl. Top with the cooked salmon, radishes, snap peas, and green onions. Sprinkle the salad with the parsley. Serve with your favorite Elimination Diet phase 2 salad dressing (see pages 271 to 276).

Yield: 2 to 4 servings

Phase 3 VARIATION

Top the salad with roasted walnuts during the nut challenge in phase 3.

SUMMER SALAD WITH BLUEBERRY VINAIGRETTE

Phase 2 *Elimination*

You can make this salad even if it's not summer! Use frozen blueberries in the dressing and any type of phase 2 fruit, such as sliced apples or pears, for the salad.

SALAD

1 head red-leaf lettuce, torn, rinsed, and spun dry

1 peach, pitted and sliced

1 avocado, sliced

½ small red onion, sliced into thin rounds

½ cup raw pumpkin seeds, toasted

DRESSING

½ cup extra-virgin olive oil

⅓ cup fresh or frozen blueberries

3 to 4 tablespoons raw coconut vinegar

1 tablespoon raw honey

½ teaspoon sea salt

To make the salad, place all the ingredients for the salad in a large bowl, toss together, and set aside.

To make the dressing, place all the ingredients in a blender and purée for about 30 seconds until smooth. Pour into a jar for serving and storing.

Serve the salad with the dressing alongside. Store any unused dressing in a sealed glass jar in the refrigerator for up to a week.

Yield: 4 to 6 servings

Phase 3 **VARIATION**

Replace the pumpkin seeds with raw walnuts that have been lightly roasted in the oven during phase 3 when you are challenging nuts.

ROASTED DELICATA SQUASH SALAD WITH APPLES AND TOASTED PUMPKIN SEEDS

Phase 2 *Elimination*

Delicata squash are a smaller, sweet winter squash with thin skin—so they don't need to be peeled before roasting or eating. Winter squash are available early to mid fall and can usually be found through March in most grocery stores. Serve this salad with a hearty bean soup or with baked salmon for a balanced meal. Top with your favorite phase 2 salad dressing recipe from pages 271 to 276.

SQUASH

1 medium delicata squash

1 tablespoon extra-virgin olive oil

¼ teaspoon sea salt

SALAD

1 head leaf lettuce or arugula, torn, rinsed, and spun dry

1 small Granny Smith apple, cored and thinly sliced

2 to 3 green onions, sliced into thin rounds

½ cup raw pumpkin seeds, toasted

¼ cup dried currants or raisins

Preheat the oven to 400°F. Line a baking sheet with parchment paper.

Rinse any dirt or debris off the squash, then cut it in half lengthwise. Scoop out the seeds with a spoon. Then place one of the squash halves on a cutting board, flesh-side down. Cut the squash into ¾-inch-thick slices (they should look like crescent moons). Repeat with second squash half. Place them on the prepared baking sheet and add the oil and salt; toss together, then spread out the pieces so they are in a single layer. Bake for 25 to 30 minutes, or until tender. Let cool completely before adding to the salad.

Place the lettuce in a large salad bowl and add the remaining ingredients along with the cooled roasted squash. Serve with your favorite phase 2 salad dressing (pages 271 to 276).

Yield: about 6 servings

NAPA CABBAGE SALAD WITH GINGER-CILANTRO DRESSING

Phase 2 *Elimination*

Low FODMAP

Serve this simple salad with some grilled chicken or salmon for a quick lunch or dinner. We like to serve it with the Chicken Fried Cauliflower "Rice" (page 260). Omit the garlic in the dressing if you are following the Low FODMAP variation of the diet.

SALAD

1 small head napa cabbage, thinly
   sliced
2 large carrots, grated
4 to 5 green onions, sliced into thin
   rounds
¼ to ½ cup raw pumpkin seeds,
   toasted

OPTIONAL ADDITIONS

diced cucumbers
thinly sliced red cabbage
sliced grilled chicken breast

DRESSING

⅓ cup extra-virgin olive oil
3 tablespoons raw coconut vinegar
1 to 2 teaspoons raw honey or pure
   maple syrup
1 (2-inch) piece fresh ginger
1 to 2 garlic cloves (optional)
½ teaspoon sea salt
small handful fresh cilantro

To make the salad, place all the ingredients in a large bowl and toss together. Top with any optional additions.

To make the dressing, place the oil, vinegar, honey, ginger, garlic, if using, and salt in a blender and purée until smooth. Then add the cilantro and blend on low speed until combined.

Serve the salad in individual portions and drizzle the dressing over each—this way, you can store any leftover salad in the refrigerator without it getting soggy from the dressing. Store any leftover dressing in a small glass jar in the refrigerator for up to 10 days.

Yield: about 6 servings

TIP

To toast pumpkin seeds, heat a 10-inch stainless steel skillet over medium heat. Add the pumpkin seeds and keep them moving in the pan. After a few minutes they should begin to puff up and turn slightly golden. If they get too dark it means the heat is too high. Remove from the pan and place on a plate to cool before adding to the salad.

CRUNCHY ROMAINE SALAD WITH ITALIAN HERB DRESSING

Phase 2 *Elimination*

Use this salad as a base and add your favorite vegetables, grilled chicken breasts, cooked fish, or cooked beans.

SALAD

1 head romaine lettuce, chopped
4 to 5 green onions, sliced into thin rounds
4 to 5 small radishes, sliced
1 medium cucumber, diced
1 large carrot, grated
1 large avocado, sliced
¼ to ½ cup raw sunflower seeds, toasted

DRESSING

¼ cup raw apple cider vinegar
2 to 3 teaspoons raw honey
2 garlic cloves (optional)
½ teaspoon sea salt
½ teaspoon freshly ground black pepper
½ cup extra-virgin olive oil
1 small handful fresh basil
1 small handful fresh parsley
1 tablespoon fresh oregano leaves

To make the salad, place the lettuce in a large bowl and top with the remaining salad ingredients.

To make the dressing, place the vinegar, honey, garlic, if using, salt, and pepper in a blender and purée until smooth. Then add the oil and fresh herbs; blend on low speed until just combined.

Serve the salad in individual portions and drizzle each with the dressing—this way, you can store any leftover salad in the refrigerator without it getting soggy from the dressing. Store any leftover dressing in a small glass jar in the refrigerator for up to 10 days.

Yield: about 6 servings

TIP

To toast sunflower seeds, heat a 10-inch stainless steel skillet over medium heat. Add the seeds and keep them moving in the pan. After a few minutes they should turn slightly golden and have a rich, fragrant smell. If they get too dark it means the heat is too high. Remove from the pan and place on a plate to cool before adding to the salad.

Phase 3 # VARIATION

Add diced red bell pepper and sliced fresh tomatoes to the salad when challenging nightshades in phase 3.

RAW KALE SALAD WITH LEMON AND GARLIC

Phase 3 *Reintroduction (citrus)*

This is one of our favorite ways to prepare raw kale! We serve it with everything from baked chicken or fish to pizza and hearty bean soups. It's even great the next day as leftovers—the kale will soften the longer it sits in the dressing, which makes it more tender and easier to chew.

1 large bunch curly kale

2 to 3 carrots, grated

¼ cup extra-virgin olive oil

zest and juice of 1 large lemon

2 garlic cloves, crushed

¼ to ½ teaspoon Herbamare or
sea salt

OPTIONAL ADDITIONS

sliced grilled chicken breast

diced avocado

dried currants or raisins

toasted pumpkin seeds

toasted sunflower seeds

hemp seeds

Remove the tough ribs that run down the center of each kale leaf, then tear the kale into pieces. Rinse in a colander and drain well, or spin dry in a salad spinner. Place the kale in a large bowl.

Add the remaining ingredients, except for any optional additions, and toss together. Let the salad rest for about 10 minutes before serving, and then toss again. Top with any optional additions just before serving.

Yield: about 6 servings

GARLIC CHICKEN SALAD

Phase 2 *Elimination*

Serve this simple, nutritious salad with Baked Winter Squash (page 243) and toasted sunflower seeds for a balanced meal. Use the Zucchini-Dill Vinaigrette (page 276), or if you are in phase 3, try the Lemon-Garlic Dressing (page 271).

CHICKEN

2 organic chicken breasts

2 garlic cloves, crushed

1 tablespoon extra-virgin olive oil

sea salt and freshly ground black
pepper

SALAD

1 head green-leaf lettuce, torn,
rinsed, and spun dry

1 cucumber, sliced

1 handful broccoli or radish sprouts

To make the chicken, heat a 10- to 12-inch cast-iron skillet over medium-low to medium heat. Pound the chicken breasts using a meat tenderizer until they are about half of their original thickness. This makes the meat more tender and helps it to cook faster in a skillet without drying out.

Place the chicken breasts in a bowl and add the remaining ingredients. Toss to coat. Place the chicken in the hot skillet; cook for 6 to 8 minutes on each side. Exact timing will depend on the thickness of the meat. Transfer the chicken to a plate or cutting board and slice into strips.

To make the salad, place the lettuce in a bowl; add the cucumber, sprouts, and sliced chicken. Serve with your favorite Elimination Diet–friendly dressing (pages 271 to 276).

Yield: 2 to 4 servings

TIP

Make up a double batch of the chicken and keep it in a glass storage container in your refrigerator to use in simple meals throughout the week.

CUCUMBER-MINT SALAD

Phase 2 *Elimination*

Our children adore this lively, fresh salad. Of course, cucumbers are their favorite vegetable! Serve this simple salad with baked chicken, fish, rice, or beans.

4 medium cucumbers, chopped	2 tablespoons raw coconut vinegar
½ cup finely diced red onion	2 tablespoons extra-virgin olive oil
½ cup chopped fresh mint	¼ to ½ teaspoon Herbamare or sea
½ cup chopped fresh parsley	salt

Place all the ingredients in a large bowl and toss together. Serve immediately.

Yield: 6 servings

RAW CAULIFLOWER, LEMON, AND LEEK SALAD

Phase 3 *Reintroduction (citrus)*

Serve this light and zesty salad with baked fish or chicken. It is also tasty over a pile of lettuce leaves and topped with toasted pine nuts.

2 small heads cauliflower, cut into florets	½ teaspoon lemon zest
1 small leek, chopped	¼ cup freshly squeezed lemon juice
½ cup chopped fresh parsley	3 tablespoons extra-virgin olive oil
	¼ teaspoon Herbamare or sea salt

Place all the ingredients in a large bowl and toss together. Serve immediately.

Yield: 6 servings

GARLIC-BRAISED COLLARD GREENS

Phase 2 *Elimination*

This is one of our "fast food" recipes. You can create a very quick meal using dark leafy greens, steamed sweet potatoes or squash, and wild fish or organic chicken. These greens also make a great addition to any breakfast—try adding cooked red beans to the collards while they are braising, then serve over cooked quinoa or rice.

1 to 2 tablespoons extra-virgin olive oil	½ to 1 cup Chicken Stock (page 295)
2 bunches collard greens, chopped	½ teaspoon sea salt or Herbamare
4 to 5 garlic cloves, crushed	

Heat the oil in a deep 11- to 12-inch skillet over medium heat. Add the collard greens and garlic; sauté for a few minutes. Then add the chicken stock. Cover and simmer for 5 to 10 minutes, or until tender. Season with sea salt.

Yield: about 4 servings

SAUTÉED KALE WITH SHIITAKE MUSHROOMS

Phase 2 *Elimination*

We make this quick vegetable dish quite often and like to serve it with baked salmon, roasted chicken, or adzuki beans and quinoa.

2 tablespoons extra-virgin olive oil or coconut oil
10 to 12 shiitake mushrooms, sliced

1 large bunch curly kale, chopped
¼ teaspoon Herbamare or sea salt
2 tablespoons water

Heat the oil in a large skillet over medium heat. Add the mushrooms and sauté for about 5 minutes. Then add the kale, Herbamare, and water; sauté for about 5 minutes more. Taste and add more salt if necessary. Serve.

Yield: 2 to 4 servings

BUTTERNUT SQUASH AND SAGE STUFFING

Phase 2 *Elimination*

This stuffing is made without bread! Using all whole-food ingredients, it's packed with nutrients like beta-carotene and immune-boosting compounds. I like to make sure the squash is cut into smaller cubes that are all about the same size, which allows for even cooking. To quickly mince the mushrooms, simply toss them all into a food processor fitted with the "s" blade and pulse until minced.

2 tablespoons extra-virgin olive oil
1 large red onion, diced
1 large butternut squash, peeled and diced (about 8 cups)
4 celery stalks, chopped (about 2 cups)

1 pound cremini mushrooms, minced
¼ cup chopped fresh sage
½ cup chopped fresh parsley
1 teaspoon Herbamare or sea salt
½ to 1 teaspoon freshly ground black pepper

Preheat the oven to 375°F.

Heat the oil in a deep 11- to 12-inch skillet. Add the onion; sauté for 5 to 7 minutes. Then add the squash, celery, and mushrooms; sauté for 10 minutes more, then add the sage, parsley, Herbamare, and pepper.

Pour the stuffing into a casserole dish with a lid; cover and bake for about 45 minutes, or until the squash is tender. Remove from the oven. Serve.

Yield: 8 servings

Phase 3 **VARIATION**

When testing pecans during phase 3, add ½ to 1 cup finely chopped, lightly roasted pecans to the top of the stuffing as it comes out of the oven. To lightly roast pecans, place them in a glass baking dish in a single layer. Roast at 375°F for about 15 minutes. Let cool, and then chop.

TIP

If you want to serve this as part of your holiday feast, prepare the stuffing and place it in the casserole dish (but don't bake it yet), cover, and refrigerate. About an hour before mealtime, place the casserole dish in the oven and bake for 45 minutes. Then sprinkle with the pecans.

CAULIFLOWER-PARSNIP MASH WITH FRESH HERBS

Phase 2 *Elimination*

Looking for a nightshade-free replacement to mashed potatoes? Try this creamy, delicious recipe! It pairs well with roasted chicken, gravy, and steamed green beans for a balanced meal.

1 small head cauliflower, cut into florets	2 tablespoons snipped fresh chives
2 medium parsnips, peeled and chopped	2 tablespoons minced fresh parsley
	¼ to ½ teaspoon sea salt or Herbamare
3 to 4 tablespoons coconut butter or extra-virgin olive oil	freshly ground black pepper

Place the cauliflower and parsnips in a steamer basket set over a few inches of water in a pot. Cover and steam for about 10 minutes, or until tender.

Drain the vegetables completely and place them in a food processor fitted with the "s" blade. Add the coconut butter or oil and process until creamy and smooth. Add the chives, parsley, salt, and pepper; pulse until combined. Taste and add more salt if necessary. You can either serve this as is or transfer it to an oiled casserole dish and bake at 450°F until lightly browned on top.

Yield: 6 servings

Phase 3 VARIATION

Replace the coconut butter with organic pastured butter when challenging dairy in phase 3.

ROASTED ROOT VEGETABLES

Phase 2 *Elimination*

Serve this warming dish alongside roasted chicken or fish and a large green salad. If you are new to using celeriac, you are in for a great surprise—it's so delicious roasted! Celeriac, also known as celery root, has a flavor similar to celery, but with a more pronounced "earthy" taste. It looks like a knobby, round, whitish root. Oftentimes they are quite large, like the size of a mini soccer ball. Sometimes you can find them smaller, in which case, you would use a whole one in this recipe.

2 large carrots, chopped

1 large beet, peeled and diced

1 medium rutabaga, peeled and
    diced

1 large parsnip, peeled and chopped

½ large celeriac, peeled and diced

2 tablespoons extra-virgin olive oil

½ teaspoon Herbamare or sea salt

freshly ground black pepper

1 tablespoon fresh thyme leaves

Preheat the oven to 400°F. Line a baking sheet with unbleached parchment paper. Place all of the vegetables on the baking sheet. Drizzle with the olive oil. Sprinkle with the salt and pepper to taste. Toss together using your hands.

Bake for about 40 minutes, or until the vegetables are tender. The exact timing will depend on the size you cut the vegetables.

Remove from the oven and sprinkle with the thyme. Serve.

Yield: about 4 servings

ROASTED BRUSSELS SPROUTS AND CAULIFLOWER

Phase 2 *Elimination*

We like to make this recipe often, and serve it alongside baked chicken or fish, or with a big raw vegetable salad and a bowl of soup.

1 pound Brussels sprouts, trimmed

1 small head cauliflower, cut into
    florets

2 tablespoons extra-virgin olive oil

¼ teaspoon sea salt

freshly ground black pepper

1 to 2 tablespoons chopped fresh
    thyme

Preheat the oven to 400°F. Place the vegetables in a 9 x 13-inch glass baking dish. Add the oil, salt, and pepper to taste. Toss together using your hands. Place the pan in the oven and roast for 30 to 35 minutes. Sprinkle the roasted vegetables with the thyme and serve immediately.

Yield: 4 to 6 servings

COCONUT-CINNAMON ROASTED SWEET POTATOES

Phase 2 *Elimination*

This is one of my favorite recipes if I am craving something sweet. Use this recipe in lieu of dessert at the end of your meal. It also pairs well with baked black cod and steamed broccoli for a simple, satisfying meal.

---

2 medium sweet potatoes, peeled and cubed

2 tablespoons melted coconut oil

1 to 2 teaspoons ground cinnamon

½ teaspoon sea salt

Preheat the oven to 425°F.

Put the sweet potatoes, oil, cinnamon, and salt in a large baking dish or on a rimmed baking sheet and mix well to coat with the oil using your hands or a large spoon. Bake, uncovered, for 30 to 35 minutes, or until the yams are very tender.

Yield: 4 servings

BAKED WINTER SQUASH

Phase 1 *Detox*

The autumn harvest brings many varieties of winter squash, including acorn, butternut, buttercup, delicata, golden turban, Hubbard, kabocha, spaghetti, and pie pumpkins. Each has its own unique flavor and a sweetness. Try serving baked winter squash with a drizzle of extra-virgin olive oil and a few dashes of cinnamon. Blend baked winter squash with Chicken Stock (page 295) or Vegetable-Seaweed Stock (page 296) for a simple, nourishing soup to sip during the detox phase.

---

1 winter squash

Preheat the oven to 350°F.

Cut the squash in half lengthwise using a strong, sharp knife. Scoop out the stringy fibers and seeds. Set the seeds aside to roast, if desired.

Place the squash flesh-side down in a roasting pan, and add ¼ to ½ inch of water. Bake until tender. Smaller squashes may take up to 35 minutes, while larger ones, including pie pumpkins, may take 45 to 90 minutes. Test by inserting a fork; it should slide in easily and the flesh should feel soft.

Yield: 1 baked squash

TIP

Try to always keep some baked squash in your refrigerator during the first two restrictive phases of the diet. It will be your go-to snack if you have nothing else prepared. Winter squash also makes a delicious dessert when warm—simply top with coconut butter and ground cinnamon!

SALT AND PEPPER KALE CHIPS

Phase 2 *Elimination*

If you are craving something salty and crunchy, make kale chips! They are a much healthier alternative to potato chips.

1 large bunch green curly kale	⅛ to ¼ teaspoon sea salt
2 tablespoons extra-virgin olive oil	⅛ to ¼ teaspoon freshly ground black pepper

Preheat the oven to 300°F.

Rinse the kale, remove the tough spine that runs down the center of each leaf, then tear the leaf into large pieces. Either use a salad spinner to spin-dry the kale or pat it dry with a clean kitchen towel. It's important that the kale is completely dry before adding the remaining ingredients and baking.

Place the kale in a large bowl and add the oil, salt, and pepper; toss together, making sure that the oil reaches all the kale leaves. Place the kale in a single layer on one or two baking sheets.

Bake the kale for about 45 minutes, flipping the leaves after about 25 minutes. It may take less time. Start checking the kale chips after 30 minutes to see if they have crisped up, and remove them from the oven once they have.

Yield: 2 to 4 servings

BASIC BROWN RICE

Phase 2 *Elimination*

Rice with just the hull removed is brown rice. Rice with the hull, bran, and germ removed is white rice. There is a wide variety of brown rice to choose from: Short grain, long grain, sweet, jasmine, and basmati are just a few. Soak brown rice overnight in a bowl of filtered water with 1 tablespoon apple cider vinegar to improve digestibility. Then rinse and drain before cooking. Soaked brown rice requires less water for cooking, so use 1½ to 1¾ cups water per cup of soaked brown rice. We like to use sprouted brown rice, which is even easier to digest than soaked rice. You can often purchase this online; see the Resources section on page 303.

1 cup brown rice	pinch sea salt
1½ to 2 cups water	

Place the rice, water, and salt in a medium pot with a tight-fitting lid and bring to a boil. Reduce the heat to a low simmer, cover, and cook for about 45 minutes, or until all of the water has been absorbed.

Never stir the rice while it is cooking. Remove the rice from the heat and let stand in the pot, covered, for about 10 minutes.

Yield: 2½ to 3½ cups

BASIC WILD RICE

Phase 2 *Elimination*

Wild rice is the seed of a grass that grows in small lakes and slow-flowing streams, and is native to North America. Native Americans harvested wild rice by canoeing into a stand of plants and bending the ripe grain heads with wooden sticks, called knockers, to get the rice into the canoe. Wild rice is closely related to true rice, as both share the same plant tribe, Oryzeae. Wild rice is higher in protein than regular brown rice and contains a high amount of zinc. Cooked wild rice can be added to soups, made into grain pilafs, or stuffed into cooked winter squash.

1 cup wild rice	pinch sea salt
2 to 2½ cups water	

Rinse the wild rice in a fine-mesh strainer, then transfer to a medium pot, add the water and sea salt, cover, and bring to a boil. Reduce the heat to low and simmer for 60 to 75 minutes.

Remove the pot from the heat and let stand, covered, for 10 minutes.

Yield: 4 cups

BASIC QUINOA

Phase 2 *Elimination*

Quinoa, pronounced "KEEN-wah," comes from the Andes Mountains in South America where it was once a staple food for the Incas. Quinoa contains all eight essential amino acids and has a delicious, light, nutty flavor. Quinoa makes wonderful grain salads and is great served with a vegetable-bean stew. Soak the quinoa overnight in a bowl of filtered water with 1 tablespoon apple cider vinegar to improve digestibility. Then rinse and drain before cooking. Soaked quinoa requires less water for cooking, so use about 1½ cups water per cup of soaked quinoa.

1 cup quinoa	pinch sea salt
1¾ cups water	

Rinse the quinoa well with warm water and drain in a fine-mesh strainer. Quinoa has a natural saponin coating that repels insects and birds. It has a bitter taste and can cause some digestive upset when consumed. Rinsing with warm water removes the saponin.

Place the rinsed quinoa, water, and salt in a medium pot with a tight-fitting lid and bring to a boil. Reduce the heat to low, cover, and simmer for 15 to 20 minutes, or until all of the water has been absorbed.

Fluff with a fork before serving.

Yield: 3 cups

ADZUKI BEAN AND RICE SALAD

Phase 2 *Elimination*

Serve this grain-and-bean salad over fresh lettuce leaves, or place a spoonful of salad in each leaf and eat it "wrap style."

SALAD

4 cups cooked long-grain brown rice

3 cups cooked adzuki beans

2 to 3 large carrots, sliced into thin rounds

1 small bunch red radishes, sliced into thin rounds

3 to 4 green onions, sliced into rounds

½ cup chopped fresh cilantro

DRESSING

5 tablespoons extra-virgin olive oil

3 tablespoons raw coconut vinegar or apple cider vinegar

2 to 3 teaspoons raw honey

½ to 1 teaspoon sea salt or Herbamare

1 to 2 garlic cloves

1 (1-inch) piece fresh ginger

lettuce leaves, for serving

To make the salad, place all the ingredients for the salad in a large bowl. Set aside.

To make the dressing, place all the ingredients in a blender and purée until smooth.

Pour the dressing over the salad and toss together. Serve over lettuce leaves. The salad can be stored in an airtight container in the refrigerator for up to 5 days.

Yield: about 6 servings

BASIL-RADISH-QUINOA SALAD

Phase 2 *Elimination*

Low FODMAP

This recipe makes a perfect, light, energizing lunch. We like to top it with leftover baked salmon or chicken and pack it in stainless steel to-go containers for busy workdays. To cook quinoa, measure 2 cups quinoa, and reference page 247 for directions.

SALAD
6 cups cooked quinoa
1 bunch red radishes, sliced
2 large carrots, diced
4 green onions, sliced into thin
  rounds

DRESSING
1 cup fresh basil leaves
½ cup extra-virgin olive oil
3 tablespoons raw coconut vinegar
1 garlic clove, peeled
1 teaspoon Herbamare or sea salt

To make the salad, place all the ingredients for the salad in a large mixing bowl.

To make the dressing, place all the ingredients for the dressing in a blender and blend on high until smooth and creamy. The dressing will be a beautiful bright green.

Pour the dressing over the salad and toss together. Serve.

Yield: 6 to 8 servings

QUINOA-CUCUMBER-DILL SALAD

Phase 3 *Reintroduction (citrus)*

Low FODMAP

Use this refreshing quinoa salad during phase 3 when you challenge lemons and limes. Add cooked beans or meat for extra protein and nutrients, if desired.

SALAD

6 to 8 cups cooked quinoa

1 large cucumber, diced

4 green onions, sliced into thin rounds

⅓ cup chopped fresh dill

DRESSING

1 teaspoon finely grated lemon zest

6 tablespoons freshly squeezed lemon juice

¼ cup extra-virgin olive oil

1 teaspoon Herbamare or sea salt

OPTIONAL ADDITIONS

2 cups cooked chickpeas

2 cups chopped cooked chicken

2 cups chopped napa cabbage

Place all of the ingredients for the salad in a large mixing bowl along with any optional additions you desire, and toss together. Whisk together the ingredients for the dressing in a small bowl and then add to the salad. Toss again. Serve.

Yield: 6 to 8 servings

VEGETABLE AND RICE NORI ROLLS

Phase 2 *Elimination*

Nori is a sea vegetable that has been dried and made into flat thin sheets. We like to spread cooked brown rice, quinoa, or seed pâtés onto it and then add a variety of vegetables. Serve with coconut aminos, wasabi, and pickled ginger, if you like. If you use wasabi, be sure to find a powder that does not contain any dyes or preservatives.

1 cup sweet brown rice	1 avocado, sliced into thin strips
½ cup short-grain brown rice	2 green onions, sliced into thin strips
3 cups water	½ cup thinly sliced red cabbage
¼ teaspoon sea salt	coconut aminos
nori sheets	wasabi
2 carrots, cut into thin matchsticks	

Place both kinds of rice in a pot with the water and sea salt. Cover, bring to a boil, then reduce the heat to low and simmer for 45 minutes. Remove from the heat and let stand, covered, for 20 minutes.

Place a sheet of nori, shiny-side down, on a clean surface. Spread a thin layer of rice to 2 inches below the top of the sheet. Place the vegetables on top of the rice at the bottom of the sheet. Tightly roll from the vegetable end. Seal the nori by wetting your finger with a little water and running it along the seam side.

Repeat this process until you have the desired amount of rolls. When ready to serve, slice the nori rolls crosswise into about 1-inch pieces with a serrated knife that has been dipped in water.

Serve with small bowls of coconut aminos and wasabi for dipping.

Yield: about 4 servings

Phase 3 **VARIATION**

When challenging soy in phase 3, add strips of sautéed organic firm tofu to the rolls alongside the vegetables. Use organic wheat-free tamari as a dipping sauce.

MUNG BEAN AND RICE KITCHEREE

Phase 2 *Elimination*

Kitcheree is a stew-like Indian meal made from mung beans and brown rice. Spices and vegetables make up the remaining ingredients and the combinations can vary widely. I use carrots, kale, peas, and cilantro, though you can use whatever vegetables you have on hand.

2 tablespoons extra-virgin olive oil

2 to 3 tablespoons finely chopped fresh ginger

1 tablespoon black mustard seeds

1 tablespoon cumin seeds

2 cups dry mung beans

2 cups short-grain brown rice

3 to 4 large carrots, cut into large chunks

1½ teaspoons turmeric powder

½ teaspoon ground coriander

10 cups water

4 cups finely chopped kale

1 to 2 cups fresh or frozen peas

½ cup chopped fresh cilantro

2 to 3 teaspoons sea salt or Herbamare

chilled coconut milk, for garnish

Heat the oil in a 6- to 8-quart pot over medium heat. Add the ginger, mustard seeds, and cumin seeds; sauté until the seeds begin to pop.

Add the mung beans, rice, carrots, turmeric, and coriander. Stir the mixture a bit so the spices evenly coat the rice and beans. Add the water and bring the stew to a boil, cover, and reduce the heat to low; simmer for about 45 minutes.

Add the kale, peas, cilantro, and salt; gently stir. Turn off the heat, cover, and let stand for about 5 minutes. Add more salt and seasonings if necessary. Dollop chilled coconut milk onto individual portions before serving, if desired.

Yield: 6 to 8 servings

MOROCCAN-SPICED VEGETABLE STEW

Phase 2 *Elimination*

Serve this warming stew over cooked quinoa, brown rice, or just as is! Add chicken or chickpeas for extra protein and nutrients. Replace some of the vegetables with others if desired. Try green beans, zucchini, or broccoli!

1 tablespoon extra-virgin olive oil or coconut oil

1 small onion, chopped

1 teaspoon Herbamare or sea salt

1 teaspoon turmeric powder

1 teaspoon ground coriander

1 teaspoon ground cardamom

½ teaspoon ground cumin

½ teaspoon freshly ground black pepper

1 (13.5-ounce) can organic coconut milk

1 cup water or Chicken Stock (page 295)

1 small head cauliflower, cut into florets

2 carrots, peeled and chopped

1 large sweet potato, peeled and chopped

1 cup fresh or frozen peas

2 cups chopped fresh spinach or kale

½ cup chopped fresh cilantro

OPTIONAL ADDITIONS

cooked chickpeas

chopped cooked chicken breast

Heat the oil in a 6-quart pot over medium heat. Add the onion and sauté for about 5 minutes, then add the Herbamare, turmeric, coriander, cardamom, cumin, and pepper; sauté a minute more. Then add the coconut milk, water, cauliflower, carrots, and sweet potato. Cover and simmer for about 10 minutes, or until the vegetables are tender.

Add the peas and spinach or kale, as well as any optional additions, and simmer for 2 minutes more. Remove from the heat and stir in the cilantro. Taste and adjust the salt and spices, if desired.

Yield: about 6 servings

Phase 3 **VARIATION**

When challenging nightshades in phase 3, add 1 cup chopped fresh tomatoes to the stew. Replace the sweet potato with 2 medium yellow or red potatoes. Add 1 teaspoon curry powder.

CHICKPEA CURRY WITH POTATOES AND KALE

Phase 3 *Reintroduction (nightshades)*

Use this recipe to challenge nightshades in phase 3. Feel free to vary the vegetables in this simple curry recipe. Try chopped zucchini, red bell peppers, cauliflower, or sweet potatoes. Just keep in mind that cooking time might vary with different vegetables—zucchini, peppers, and cauliflower take considerably less time to cook than carrots and potatoes. Serve the stew over cooked brown rice or quinoa. We like to serve sliced raw cucumbers on the side as well.

2 tablespoons coconut oil or extra-virgin olive oil	4 medium yellow or red potatoes, chopped
1 small onion, chopped	3 cups cooked chickpeas
1 jalapeño pepper, finely chopped	3 cups water
1 tablespoon black mustard seeds	¼ cup tomato paste
1 tablespoon curry powder	1 small bunch kale, chopped
1½ to 2 teaspoons sea salt	½ cup chopped fresh cilantro
4 large carrots, chopped	

Heat the oil in a 6-quart pot over medium heat. Add the onion and sauté for 5 to 7 minutes. Then add the jalapeño, mustard seeds, curry powder, and salt; sauté for a few minutes more.

Add the carrots, potatoes, chickpeas, water, and tomato paste; cover and simmer for about 15 minutes, or until the vegetables are tender. Add the kale and cilantro; simmer for a few minutes more. Taste and adjust the salt or seasonings, if desired.

Yield: 8 servings

VARIATION

If your digestive system cannot tolerate legumes, then replace the chickpeas with 1 to 1½ pounds chopped cooked organic chicken breast or thigh meat.

BLACK BEAN, YAM, AND AVOCADO TACOS

Phase 2 *Elimination*

Use our simple Brown Rice Tortilla recipe (page 223) as the wrap for these tacos. You can also try using a large collard green, cabbage leaf, or lettuce leaf.

2 cups cooked black beans, drained
few pinches sea salt (optional)
1 large yam, cooked
1 large avocado, mashed

lettuce or arugula leaves
4 Brown Rice Tortillas (page 223)

GARNISH
chopped cilantro

Place the cooked black beans in a serving bowl and sprinkle with salt, if desired. Peel the cooked yam, place the flesh in a separate serving bowl, and mash it with a fork. Place the mashed avocado in a separate serving bowl. Set the lettuce leaves and tortillas on a platter.

Let each person assemble his or her own taco. Garnish with chopped cilantro.

Yield: 4 servings

> **TIP**
>
> To cook a yam, leave the skin on, prick it with a fork, place it in a small baking dish, and bake for about 1 hour at 350°F. Alternatively, you can cook the yam on the stove by steaming it—leave the skin on, slice the yam into thick slices, place them in a small pot, and fill it with an inch or two of water. Cover and cook for about 15 minutes, or until the yam slices are soft; drain, remove the peels, and mash.

POACHED SALMON WITH SUMMER VEGETABLES

Phase 3 *Reintroduction (nightshades)*

This is one of our favorite quick and easy meals. Serve it alongside a big salad and possibly some cooked quinoa or quinoa-rice noodles, and you will have a beautiful, nourishing, Elimination Diet meal.

2 tablespoons extra-virgin olive oil

1 small red onion, halved and cut into half-moons

1 fennel bulb, halved and cut into half-moons

2 medium zucchini, sliced on an angle into ½-inch pieces

4 to 5 plum tomatoes, chopped

1½ to 2 pounds wild salmon fillets

1 to 2 teaspoons Italian seasoning

½ teaspoon sea salt or Herbamare

freshly ground black pepper

½ cup water or Chicken Stock (page 295)

¼ cup finely chopped fresh parsley

¼ cup finely chopped fresh basil

Heat the oil in a deep 11- or 12-inch skillet over medium heat. Add the onion and sauté for about 5 minutes. Then add the fennel, zucchini, and tomatoes; sauté for 3 to 4 minutes more. Push the vegetables to the sides of the pan.

Add the salmon fillets. Sprinkle the Italian seasoning, salt, and pepper over the salmon fillets. Pour the water into the pan. Cover and simmer for 10 to 15 minutes. Exact timing will depend on the thickness of your salmon fillets. I suggest checking them at 8 minutes for doneness. Be careful not to overcook them! Sprinkle the parsley and basil over the salmon and vegetables. Serve.

Yield: 4 to 6 servings

(Low FODMAP) **VARIATION**

Omit the red onion in this recipe. Instead, garnish the finished dish with snipped fresh chives or chopped green onions.

HERB-ROASTED WILD SALMON

Phase 2 *Elimination*

Low FODMAP

Use this recipe during phases 2 and 3 of the diet—the healthy omega-3 oils in the salmon will help to calm down any inflammation in the body. This is our go-to "fast food" meal when I'm out of time and dinner needs to get on the table quickly. Serve with steamed yams or Baked Winter Squash (page 243) along with either sautéed dark leafy greens or a large raw salad.

---

2 to 2½ pounds skin-on wild salmon fillets

¼ cup chopped fresh herbs (lemon thyme, dill, parsley, oregano, rosemary)

½ teaspoon sea salt or Herbamare

freshly ground black pepper

2 tablespoons extra-virgin olive oil

Preheat the oven to 400°F. Line a 9 x 13-inch baking dish with unbleached parchment paper (this is optional, but makes cleanup really easy).

Place the salmon skin-side down in the baking dish. Evenly sprinkle the herbs over the salmon. Sprinkle with the salt and pepper. Drizzle the olive oil over the salmon and herbs.

Bake for 10 minutes per inch of salmon fillet thickness. A thick cut of king salmon will usually take about 20 minutes, while sockeye only needs about

8 minutes. Salmon will continue to cook after you remove it from the oven so it is best to underestimate the cooking time needed.

Yield: about 6 servings

TIP

Leftover salmon makes a great addition to your breakfast or lunch. Use it to top sautéed greens stuffed inside of a baked yam or on top of a large green salad.

Phase 3 **VARIATION**

Add fresh lemon slices on top of the salmon before baking when challenging citrus in phase 3.

BAKED SALMON WITH CASHEW-GINGER SAUCE

Phase 3 *Reintroduction (cashews)*

Use this recipe during phase 3 when you are challenging cashews. If you can't find raw cashew butter, you can use ⅓ cup raw cashews soaked in water for about 1 hour (and then drained). Use raw pumpkin seed butter in place of the cashew butter during phase 2. Serve with Sautéed Kale with Shiitake Mushrooms (page 239) and steamed sweet potatoes for a simple, nourishing meal.

1½ pounds wild salmon fillets
1 tablespoon coconut oil
Herbamare or sea salt

SAUCE
¼ cup raw cashew butter
¼ cup water

3 tablespoons coconut aminos
1 tablespoon raw coconut vinegar
1 (1-inch) piece fresh ginger
1 garlic clove, peeled

Preheat the oven to 400°F. Place the salmon fillet in a small baking dish. Rub the coconut oil on the top of the fish, then sprinkle with Herbamare. Bake for 10 minutes per inch of thickness, 10 to 20 minutes depending on the size of the fillet.

While the fish is cooking, place all the ingredients for the sauce in a blender and blend until smooth. Pour the sauce into a small saucepan and heat over very low heat until thickened and warm. Add more water for a thinner sauce. Drizzle the sauce over the cooked fish fillet and serve immediately.

Yield: 3 to 4 servings

Phase 3 **VARIATION**

Replace the coconut aminos with organic wheat-free tamari when challenging soy.

TIP

We prefer to purchase wild Alaskan troll-caught king salmon, as it is one of the most sustainable forms of salmon and also has the least amount of environmental toxins. Always look for wild Pacific salmon; never buy farmed or Atlantic salmon.

POMEGRANATE CHICKEN TACOS

Phase 2 *Elimination*

This recipe is designed for your slow cooker and takes just minutes to prepare! You can put it together in the morning, then set your slow cooker to low, and you will have a meal ready when you get home from work. Use the Brown Rice Tortillas (page 223) or fresh collard greens for your taco shells.

CHICKEN

1½ pounds organic skinless, boneless chicken breasts or thighs

1 cup pure pomegranate juice

1 small onion, halved and cut into half-moons

2 to 3 garlic cloves, crushed

1 tablespoon extra-virgin olive oil

2 teaspoons ground cumin

2 teaspoons Herbamare or sea salt

½ to 1 teaspoon freshly ground black pepper

TACOS

Brown Rice Tortillas (page 223) or collard green leaves

thinly sliced napa cabbage or romaine lettuce

sliced avocado

shredded cucumber

To make the chicken, place all the ingredients for the chicken in a 3-quart slow cooker. Cover and cook on low for 7 to 8 hours, or on high for 3 to 4 hours. Remove the chicken from the slow cooker and place it on a plate. Use two forks to shred the chicken, then place the shredded chicken back in the slow cooker and mix it into the cooked onions and juices. Let it cook uncovered, for 10 to 15 minutes more.

To assemble the tacos, place a scoop of the shredded chicken into the center of each tortilla, then add a small handful of napa cabbage, a few slices of avocado, and a spoonful of shredded cucumber.

Yield: about 4 servings

TIP

Make sure to purchase pure pomegranate juice with no other juices or sweeteners added. We buy organic Just Pomegranate juice by R.W. Knudsen.

CHICKEN FRIED CAULIFLOWER "RICE"

Phase 2 *Elimination*

Pulsing a whole head of raw cauliflower into small pieces in a food processor can replicate white rice. This nutrient-dense, vegetable-rich meal is great for breakfast, lunch, or dinner. Serve it with Napa Cabbage Salad with Ginger-Cilantro Dressing (page 232).

1 medium head cauliflower, coarsely chopped

2 tablespoons extra-virgin olive oil or coconut oil

½ white onion, diced

2 large carrots, diced

2 celery stalks, diced

2 teaspoons grated fresh ginger

½ pound organic skinless, boneless chicken breasts or thighs, chopped

5 to 6 shiitake mushrooms, sliced

1 small zucchini, diced

1 cup fresh or frozen peas

2 cups sliced napa cabbage

3 tablespoons coconut aminos

½ teaspoon sea salt

¼ teaspoon freshly ground white pepper

GARNISHES

sliced green onions

chopped fresh cilantro

Place the chopped cauliflower in a food processor fitted with the "s" blade. Pulse until the cauliflower is broken down into tiny, rice-like pieces, and set aside.

Heat the oil in a deep 11- to 12-inch skillet over medium heat. Add the onion, carrots, celery, and ginger; sauté for about 5 minutes. Then add the chicken and sauté for a few minutes more. Next add the mushrooms and zucchini; sauté for 2 minutes more.

Add the minced cauliflower and stir it into the chicken-vegetable mixture; sauté for about 7 minutes. Add the peas, napa cabbage, coconut aminos, salt, and white pepper; sauté for another few minutes. Taste and adjust the salt and seasonings, if desired. Garnish each serving with sliced green onions and cilantro.

Yield: 4 to 6 servings

CHICKEN AND VEGETABLE STIR-FRY

Phase 2 *Elimination*

Try this tasty soy-free stir-fry served over sprouted brown rice or cooked spaghetti squash. I prefer to use a 12-inch cast-iron skillet to cook the chicken—it cooks evenly and quickly this way without burning. Never use any type of nonstick cookware because of the chemicals the nonstick coating contains!

CHICKEN	STIR-FRY
1 to 1½ pounds organic skinless, boneless chicken breasts, thinly sliced	2 tablespoons coconut oil for cooking
¼ cup coconut aminos	1 small onion, halved and cut into half-moons
1 tablespoon coconut vinegar	3 to 4 cups sliced savoy cabbage
2 to 3 garlic cloves, crushed	2 to 3 cups broccoli florets
1 tablespoon grated fresh ginger	
¼ teaspoon sea salt	

To make the chicken, place all the ingredients for the chicken in a small mixing bowl. Let it marinate on the counter for about 20 minutes or in the refrigerator for up to 4 hours.

To make the stir-fry, heat 1 tablespoon of the coconut oil in an 11- or 12-inch skillet over medium-high heat. Add half of the chicken; sauté for about 4 minutes, then remove from the pan and place on a plate. Repeat with the remaining chicken.

Add the remaining 1 tablespoon coconut oil, and then add the onion and sauté for about 5 minutes. Add the cabbage and broccoli; sauté for about 5 minutes more. Then return the chicken to the pan and stir together. Add more salt and seasonings, if desired.

Yield: 4 to 6 servings

Phase 3 **VARIATION**

Replace the coconut aminos with organic wheat-free tamari when challenging soy in phase 3.

CHICKEN-SPINACH BURGERS

Phase 2 *Elimination*

Low FODMAP

This recipe can be made when you are pinched for time—it's so fast! We like to serve each burger topped with mashed avocado, sliced cucumbers, and radishes. And then we wrap each one in a piece of butter lettuce.

1 cup frozen spinach, thawed

4 green onions, cut into 1-inch pieces

1 tablespoon fresh oregano leaves

1 teaspoon Herbamare or sea salt

½ teaspoon freshly ground black pepper

1½ pounds organic skinless, boneless chicken thighs or breasts

extra-virgin olive oil or coconut oil for cooking

Squeeze out any excess liquid from the thawed spinach, then place the spinach in a food processor fitted with the "s" blade. Add the green onions, oregano, Herbamare, and pepper; pulse a few times. Then add the chicken and process until the chicken is ground and the mixture starts to form a ball. It does not take long, only about 30 seconds.

With oiled hands, form the mixture into about eight patties and set them on a plate or baking sheet. Heat about 1 tablespoon of oil in a large cast-iron skillet over medium-low heat. Add four of the patties to the pan and cook for 4 to 5 minutes on each side. Transfer the cooked patties to a plate and repeat with the remaining patties. Serve.

Yield: 8 burgers

VEGETABLE CHICKEN BAKE

Phase 2 *Elimination*

You can create a beautiful meal in no time at all with this recipe. Use the vegetables I suggest below or choose your own—try cauliflower, broccoli, green beans, parsnips, turnips, yams, Brussels sprouts, and leeks. Serve this recipe along with a large green salad and cooked quinoa.

2 organic bone-in, skin-on chicken breasts	4 to 5 thin carrots, cut into 3-inch pieces
2 organic bone-in, skin-on chicken legs	½ pound asparagus spears, trimmed
1 small onion, cut into chunks	1 to 2 teaspoons dried thyme
4 small zucchini, cut into 3-inch pieces	1 teaspoon Herbamare or sea salt
	freshly ground black pepper
	3 to 4 tablespoons extra-virgin olive oil

Preheat the oven to 400°F. Place the chicken in a 10 x 14-inch baking dish. Distribute the vegetables evenly around the chicken, putting the carrots on the bottom and the zucchini and asparagus on the top. Sprinkle everything with the thyme, salt, and pepper to taste. Drizzle the olive oil evenly over the chicken and vegetables.

Place the chicken and vegetables in the oven and roast for 35 to 40 minutes, or until the chicken juices run clear. Remove the pan from the oven and let rest on the counter for about 10 minutes. Serve slices of chicken with the roasted vegetables, and then spoon some of the pan juices onto each plate.

Yield: 6 servings

TIP

Be sure to use very thick asparagus spears. Thin spears will overcook! If you can't find thick ones, just omit the asparagus and substitute another vegetable, such as cauliflower. Also, I prefer to use tender baby carrots (not the processed baby carrots you find in the store) from my farmers' market. If you can only find mature, thick carrots, then cut them in half lengthwise first to help them cook properly—carrots generally have a longer cooking time compared to other vegetables.

WHOLE ROASTED CHICKEN WITH ROSEMARY

Phase 2 *Elimination*

Make an easy meal by roasting a whole chicken for dinner. Serve with Cauliflower-Parsnip Mash with Fresh Herbs (page 240) and steamed green beans. Use the leftover meat the next day to top a green salad. Then use the chicken bones and skin to make a nourishing stock.

1 (4- to 5-pound) whole organic chicken

2 to 3 shallots, chopped

4 to 5 garlic cloves

3 sprigs fresh rosemary, plus ¼ cup chopped fresh rosemary

½ teaspoon freshly ground black pepper

1 to 2 teaspoons sea salt

2 tablespoons extra-virgin olive oil

arrowroot powder

Preheat the oven to 425°F.

Place the chicken in a roasting pan or glass baking dish. Pat it dry. Place some of the shallots and garlic into the cavity of the chicken, and then scatter the rest around the chicken in the pan. Place the sprigs of rosemary into the cavity as well.

Sprinkle the chopped rosemary, pepper, and salt over the chicken. Drizzle the oil over the chicken as well. Add about 1 cup water to the bottom of the pan.

Roast the chicken for 25 minutes, then reduce the oven temperature to 325°F and bake for approximately 1 hour more. The chicken is done when its juices run clear or when internal temperature reaches 165°F. Exact timing will depend on the size of the chicken. Larger ones may take more time, while smaller ones will need less.

Remove the chicken from the oven and place it on a plate; let it rest for about 10 minutes before you begin carving. Pour the pan juices through a fine-mesh strainer into a small saucepan.

To make a gravy, whisk in 1 tablespoon arrowroot powder per cup of pan juices. Set the pan over medium-low heat and simmer until thickened. Season with salt and pepper to taste.

Yield: about 6 servings

SPICED CHICKEN AND YAMS

Phase 2 *Elimination*

This is another delicious option for roasting a whole chicken for dinner. The leftover meat is perfect for another meal, such as the Harvest Squash Soup (page 219), and be sure also to use the bones and skin to make a rich, healing stock. Serve this recipe along with Garlic-Braised Collard Greens (page 238) and steamed green beans for a complete meal.

1 (4- to 5-pound) whole organic chicken

1 medium onion, chopped

3 medium yams, peeled and chopped

2 tablespoons extra-virgin olive oil

3 teaspoons ground cumin

1 teaspoon ground cinnamon

½ teaspoon freshly ground black pepper

2 teaspoons sea salt

Preheat the oven to 425°F.

Place the chicken in a large pan (I use a 10 x 14-inch pan). Pat it dry. Place a small handful of the onion into the cavity of the chicken, then scatter the rest around the chicken in the pan. Nestle all of the yam pieces around the chicken over the onion. Drizzle the chicken and vegetables with the olive oil.

In a small bowl, mix together the cumin, cinnamon, pepper, and salt. Take about half of the mixture and rub it into the chicken. Sprinkle the remainder over the yams and onion; gently toss to coat.

Roast for 25 minutes, then reduce the heat to 325°F and bake for approximately 1 hour more. The chicken is done when its juices run clear or when internal temperature reaches 165°F. Exact timing will depend on the size of the chicken. Larger ones may take more time, while smaller ones will need less.

Remove the chicken from the oven and place it on a plate; let it rest for about 10 minutes before you begin carving. Serve chicken slices with the yams, onions, and pan juices.

Yield: about 6 servings

GREEK CHICKEN LETTUCE WRAPS

Phase 3 *Reintroduction (citrus, cashews)*

Use this recipe in phase 3 after you have reintroduced citrus and are working on challenging cashews. This chicken salad is made without mayonnaise, instead using a dressing made from lemon juice and creamy raw cashew butter. We like to serve it in butter lettuce leaves, but romaine or leaf lettuce works just fine!

SALAD
4 cups chopped cooked organic chicken
1 medium cucumber, chopped
½ cup finely diced red onion

DRESSING
½ cup raw cashew butter

¼ cup freshly squeezed lemon juice
¼ cup water
½ teaspoon Herbamare

OTHER INGREDIENTS
6 to 8 butter lettuce leaves
1 handful chopped fresh parsley

To make the salad, place all the ingredients for the salad in a large bowl and toss to combine.

To make the dressing, place all the ingredients for the dressing in a blender and blend on high until smooth and creamy. Pour the dressing over the salad and gently toss together.

To assemble the wraps, place a few large spoonfuls of the chicken salad onto each lettuce leaf. Sprinkle with chopped parsley. Serve.

Yield: 6 servings

TIP

To cook chicken, place 2 or 3 bone-in, skin-on organic chicken breasts in a 4-quart pot. Add 6 to 8 cups water, 1 small chopped onion, 1 chopped celery stalk, 2 teaspoons sea salt, 1 teaspoon whole black peppercorns, and a handful of fresh parsley. Cover and simmer for 30 to 40 minutes. Remove the chicken from the pot and set it on a plate to cool. Pour the stock through a fine-mesh strainer; discard the solids left in the strainer. Pour the stock into quart jars and store in your refrigerator. Use the stock to make soup. Once the chicken is cool, chop or shred it and use as directed.

BRINED TURKEY BREAST

Phase 2 *Elimination*

Brining turkey makes the meat so tender and flavorful. Once you try it this way you might never want to go back to roasting turkey without brining!

---

1 (2½- to 3-pound) bone-in, skin-on organic turkey breast

BRINE
4 cups organic apple juice
4 cups water

¼ cup sea salt
1 small onion, sliced
2 bay leaves
2 sprigs fresh rosemary
2 sprigs fresh thyme
1 teaspoon whole black peppercorns

Place the turkey breast in a large bowl or stainless steel pot. Add all of the ingredients for the brine, cover with a lid, and refrigerate for 24 to 72 hours.

When ready to cook, preheat the oven to 350°F. Set out a 9 x 13-inch glass baking dish. Remove the turkey from the brine and place it in the baking dish. I also like to remove the onions and herb sprigs from the brine and place them in the pan with the turkey.

Roast the turkey for about 2 hours, or until its juices run clear.

Yield: about 6 servings

TURKEY-HERB-QUINOA MEATBALLS

Phase 2 *Elimination*

Low FODMAP

These meatballs freeze amazingly well. I like to freeze them in serving-size containers to have a quick lunch ready to go when needed. Serve meatballs and sauce over baked spaghetti squash with a large green salad.

MEATBALLS

1 bunch green onions, coarsely chopped

1 handful fresh parsley

1 handful fresh basil

1 to 2 garlic cloves, peeled (optional)

2 cups cooked quinoa

2 pounds ground organic turkey

1 tablespoon Italian seasoning

1 to 2 teaspoons Herbamare

½ to 1 teaspoon freshly ground black pepper

extra-virgin olive oil for cooking

SAUCE

2 cups homemade turkey stock or Chicken Stock (page 295)

2 tablespoons arrowroot powder

GARNISH

chopped fresh parsley, for serving

To make the meatballs, place the green onions, parsley, basil, and garlic, if using, in a food processor fitted with the "s" blade. Process until finely ground. Then add the cooked quinoa and process again. Add the turkey, Italian seasoning, Herbamare, and pepper; process until all the ingredients are combined. You may need to pulse the mixture a few times and scrape down the sides. Using lightly oiled hands, roll the mixture into equal-size meatballs. Set them on plates as you roll them.

Heat a tablespoon or two of extra-virgin olive oil in a large skillet over medium heat. Place enough meatballs in the pan so they still have some room to move. Sauté for 5 to 10 minutes, moving the meatballs around a little so they cook on all sides. They won't be all the way cooked at this point, so don't eat them. Transfer to a clean plate. Repeat with the remaining uncooked meatballs. Add more oil in between batches, if necessary.

To make the sauce, combine the stock and arrowroot powder in a bowl and whisk together to dissolve the arrowroot. Once you have sautéed all of the meatballs, pour the sauce mixture into the pan, and add cooked meatballs back into the pan; cover and simmer on low heat for about 15 minutes. Garnish with chopped fresh parsley and serve.

Yield: about 24 meatballs

MUSTARD-HERB LAMB BURGERS

Phase 2 *Elimination*

Low FODMAP

When eliminating gluten and other grains from your diet, you can use two romaine lettuce leaves or napa cabbage leaves as your "bun" to hold your favorite fixings! Be sure to use Eden Organic mustard, as it is the only brand that uses apple cider vinegar. If you can't find this particular brand, then omit the mustard altogether, or replace it with about 1 teaspoon yellow mustard powder.

BURGERS

1 pound ground lamb

1 tablespoon stone-ground mustard

3 to 4 green onions, minced

¼ cup minced fresh herbs (dill, parsley, mint)

½ teaspoon ground cumin

½ teaspoon sea salt or Herbamare

½ teaspoon freshly ground black pepper

extra-virgin olive oil for cooking

OTHER INGREDIENTS

mustard

mashed avocado

fresh mint leaves

lettuce leaves

To make the burgers, place all the burger ingredients except for the oil in a large bowl and mix together using your hands or a large spoon. Form the mixture into four to six patties and set them on a plate.

Heat about 1 tablespoon of oil in a large cast-iron skillet over medium heat. Add the burgers one at a time. Cook for about 5 minutes on each side. Continue cooking for a few minutes more, if you would like your burgers well-done.

Spread each burger with mustard and top with mashed avocado and fresh mint leaves. Serve in between two pieces of lettuce.

Yield: 4 to 6 servings

DIPS, CONDIMENTS, SAUCES, AND DRESSINGS

HUMMUS

Phase 3 *Reintroduction (sesame)*

Hummus is a traditional Middle Eastern dish made from garbanzo beans, also called chickpeas, and tahini. It makes an excellent dip for fresh vegetables or a great spread for sandwiches or wraps.

3 cups cooked chickpeas	1 teaspoon garlic powder, or
½ cup sesame tahini	2 garlic cloves, crushed
½ cup freshly squeezed lemon juice	1 teaspoon ground cumin
¼ cup extra-virgin olive oil	1 to 2 teaspoons sea salt or
	Herbamare
	¼ cup bean cooking liquid or water

Place all the ingredients in a food processor fitted with the "s" blade and process until smooth and creamy.

You will want to taste the hummus to see if it needs more lemon, tahini, garlic, or salt. For a thinner consistency, add more water and process again. Hummus freezes very well.

Yield: 4 cups

LEMON-GARLIC DRESSING

Phase 3 *Reintroduction (citrus)*

Use this dressing to top your favorite salad or use it to top a bowl of lightly steamed vegetables.

¼ cup extra-virgin olive oil	1 to 2 garlic cloves, crushed
zest and juice of 1 lemon	¼ teaspoon sea salt

Combine all the ingredients in a small bowl and whisk together. Serve. Store any leftovers in a small glass jar in the refrigerator for up to a week.

Yield: about ½ cup

BLUEBERRY VINAIGRETTE

Phase 2 *Elimination*

Low FODMAP

This is one of our favorite Elimination Diet salad dressings . . . actually, it's one of our favorite salad dressings, period! Serve it over a baby kale salad with leftover cooked salmon, or atop a pile of crunchy romaine lettuce, toasted pumpkin seeds, and sliced avocados.

½ cup extra-virgin olive oil	2 to 3 teaspoons pure maple syrup
⅓ cup fresh or frozen blueberries	½ teaspoon sea salt
3 to 4 tablespoons raw coconut vinegar	1 tablespoon fresh lemon thyme or another fresh herb

Place all the ingredients in a blender and blend until smooth. Pour into a glass jar, cover, and refrigerate until ready to serve.

Yield: about 1 cup

GREEN GODDESS DRESSING

Phase 2 *Elimination*

This is my go-to dressing when I want something rich and creamy to top my salad. Avocados are an excellent source of monounsaturated fats and other nutrients that help the skin and hair glow. Make a double batch of this dressing to have on hand for the week.

½ small avocado	1 tablespoon raw apple cider vinegar
½ cup water	¼ teaspoon sea salt
1 garlic clove, peeled	1 small handful fresh parsley

Place all the ingredients, except for the parsley, in a blender and blend until smooth and creamy. Add the parsley and blend on low speed until combined.

Yield: about ¾ cup

Phase 3 VARIATION

Replace the apple cider vinegar with freshly squeezed lemon juice during the citrus challenge.

CREAMY GARLIC–HEMP SEED DRESSING

Phase 2 *Elimination*

Drizzle this creamy, nut-free, dairy-free dressing over your favorite green salad. I like to serve it over mixed organic baby greens with sliced avocados for a simple, nourishing salad.

½ cup hemp seeds

½ cup water

2 tablespoons raw apple cider vinegar

1 to 2 garlic cloves, peeled

½ teaspoon kelp granules

¼ teaspoon sea salt or Herbamare

OPTIONAL ADDITIONS

1 handful fresh cilantro

1 handful fresh parsley

1 handful fresh basil

Place all the ingredients in a blender (except the optional additions) and blend until smooth and creamy. Add any optional additions (my favorite is the cilantro) and blend again on low speed to incorporate.

Serve over your favorite salad. Store any leftovers in a glass jar in the refrigerator for up to a week.

Yield: about ¾ cup

CASHEW RANCH DRESSING

Phase 3 *Reintroduction (cashews, citrus)*

Use this recipe after you have already reintroduced citrus and are challenging cashews. If you found that you have a citrus sensitivity, then replace the lemon juice with 3 tablespoons raw apple cider vinegar. My favorite way to use this dressing is drizzled over a salad of crunchy romaine lettuce, cucumbers, and radishes.

½ cup raw cashews

juice of 1 large lemon (3 to 4 tablespoons)

¼ cup water

¼ cup extra-virgin olive oil

1 small garlic clove

½ teaspoon sea salt or Herbamare

¼ to ½ teaspoon freshly ground black pepper

2 tablespoons chopped fresh dill

2 tablespoons chopped fresh parsley

2 tablespoons chopped fresh chives

Place the cashews in a small bowl and cover them with about 1 inch of water. Let them soak on your kitchen counter for about 3 hours. Then drain and rinse and place them in a blender. Add all the remaining ingredients except the fresh herbs. Blend on high until smooth and creamy.

Add the fresh herbs and blend on low speed until incorporated but not completely blended. You want to have little green flecks of herbs in your white dressing—not green dressing!

Taste and adjust the salt and seasonings if needed. Pour the dressing into a glass jar with a tight-fitting lid and store in your refrigerator for up to 10 days. Once chilled, it can be used as a dip for veggies. Bring to room temperature and thin out with a few tablespoons of water if needed before using as a salad dressing.

Yield: about 1 cup

CREAMY SUNFLOWER SEED–PARSLEY DRESSING

Phase 2 *Elimination*

Use this dressing as a creamy dip for carrot sticks or cucumber slices, or drizzle it over a salad of organic lettuce, grated raw beets, grated carrots, and broccoli sprouts.

½ cup raw sunflower seeds	1 garlic clove, peeled
¼ cup water	½ teaspoon sea salt or Herbamare
3 tablespoons raw apple cider vinegar	¼ cup extra-virgin olive oil
	1 small handful fresh parsley

Soak the sunflower seeds in a small bowl of filtered water for 6 to 8 hours, or overnight. Drain and rinse the seeds and place them in a blender along with the water, vinegar, garlic, and salt. Blend until supersmooth and creamy. Then add the oil and parsley; blend on low speed until combined. Store in a glass jar in your refrigerator for up to 10 days.

Yield: about 1½ cups

GINGER-APPLE DRESSING

Phase 2 *Elimination*

Use this citrus- and vinegar-free dressing in a cabbage slaw or drizzled over your favorite salad. Be sure to use a very tart apple, such as Granny Smith. This gives the dressing a tangy flavor.

1 medium Granny Smith apple, cored and chopped	1 small garlic clove, peeled
½ cup water	1 (1-inch) piece of fresh ginger
⅓ cup extra-virgin olive oil	¼ to ½ teaspoon sea salt

Place all the ingredients in a blender and blend for about 60 seconds, or until smooth and creamy. Taste and add a little more salt if needed, and blend again.

Store the dressing in a tightly covered glass jar in the refrigerator for up to a week.

Yield: about 1½ cups

ZUCCHINI-DILL VINAIGRETTE

Phase 2 *Elimination*

Low FODMAP

Use this simple, flavorful recipe to dress Garlic Chicken Salad (page 236) or your favorite Elimination Diet salad.

½ cup chopped raw zucchini

6 tablespoons extra-virgin olive oil

3 tablespoons raw apple cider vinegar

2 teaspoons raw honey

1 teaspoon dried dill

½ teaspoon sea salt

1 garlic clove (optional)

Place all the ingredients in a blender and blend until smooth and creamy. Pour into a glass jar with a tight-fitting lid and store in the refrigerator for up to 10 days.

Yield: about 1 cup

COCONUT SOUR CREAM

Phase 2 *Elimination*

Low FODMAP

This is a great replacement for dairy sour cream—it's so simple to make! Dollop it on top of bean soups or tacos, use it as a base for herbed sour cream dips, or stir in a little honey and dollop it over fresh berries. Be sure to use full-fat coconut milk, not the light variety. For the probiotic powder, we use Klaire Labs Ther-Biotic Complete powder.

2 (13.5-ounce) cans full-fat coconut milk, chilled

1 teaspoon probiotic powder

pinch sea salt

Place the cans of coconut milk in the refrigerator for about 24 hours. Then open the cans and scoop the thick white cream at the top into a small saucepan. Pour off the water into a jar and reserve it for another use (such as for smoothies).

Heat the coconut cream over the lowest heat to about 97° to 98°F. Remove the pan from the heat and whisk in the probiotic powder. Pour the mixture into a clean quart jar and cover with a clean dishtowel secured with a rubber band.

Let the jar sit out on your kitchen counter for 24 to 48 hours to culture. Then stir in a pinch or two of sea salt, cover the jar with a lid, and refrigerate to solidify. Use as desired.

Yield: 1 to 2 cups (varies depending on how much cream is in each can)

TIP

Depending on the temperature where your coconut milk is stored, you may not need to refrigerate the cans to get the cream and water to separate. In the wintertime, my pantry is cool enough to keep the fat and water separated so I just open the cans and get started right away on this recipe.

NIGHTSHADE-FREE PASTA SAUCE

Phase 2 *Elimination*

This sauce has a texture, color, and flavor very similar to traditional pasta sauce. Use it to top baked spaghetti squash or cooked quinoa spaghetti noodles (see Resources on page 303 to find an Elimination Diet–friendly brand). You can also cook ground lamb or beef (when challenging beef) in a skillet and then add 2 to 3 cups of this sauce to the ground meat for a heartier pasta sauce.

---

2 tablespoons extra-virgin olive oil
1 small onion, chopped
4 to 5 garlic cloves, peeled and chopped
3 large carrots, peeled and chopped
1 medium beet, peeled and chopped

1 tablespoon dried Italian herbs
1½ teaspoons sea salt or Herbamare
¼ to ½ teaspoon freshly ground black pepper
3 to 4 tablespoons raw apple cider vinegar
3 cups water

Heat the oil in a 3-quart pot over medium heat. Add the onion and sauté for 5 to 10 minutes, or until soft and beginning to change color. Then add the garlic, carrots, and beet; sauté for 5 minutes more.

Add the Italian seasoning, salt, pepper, vinegar, and water. Cover and simmer for about 25 minutes, or until the vegetables are very tender. Use an immersion blender to purée the sauce in the pan, or carefully transfer the sauce to a blender and blend until very smooth. Taste and add more salt and pepper, if desired. Also, if you would like more tang, add extra apple cider vinegar, 1 to 2 teaspoons at a time until the sauce is at your desired acidity.

Yield: about 1 quart

TIP

Be sure to only use Italian seasoning that contains just dried herbs. Some brands can contain dried onion, red peppers, or lemon peel, which are not safe during the first two phases of the diet.

FRESH BERRIES WITH WHIPPED VANILLA COCONUT CREAM

Phase 2 *Elimination*

Low FODMAP

Use this simple recipe as a replacement for whipped heavy cream. The coconut cream will begin to soften as it sits at room temperature and will soften quickly on a hot summer afternoon, so be sure to keep it chilled. You can easily rewhip it after you remove the container from the refrigerator.

WHIPPED VANILLA COCONUT CREAM

2 (14.5-ounce) cans full-fat coconut milk, chilled for 12 hours

1 to 2 tablespoons coconut nectar, honey, or pure maple syrup

½ to 1 teaspoon raw vanilla powder

pinch sea salt

BERRIES

2 pints fresh organic berries (raspberries, blueberries, strawberries)

To make the whipped vanilla coconut cream, open the chilled cans of coconut milk and scoop the thick white coconut cream from the top into a mixing bowl. Pour the watery milk into a jar and reserve to use in your favorite fruit smoothie.

Add the liquid sweetener, vanilla, and salt to the bowl with the coconut cream. Using an electric mixer, whip the chilled cream to soft peaks. Divide the berries among six small bowls and dollop with the whipped coconut cream. Serve immediately.

Yield: 6 servings

VANILLA-COCONUT SNOWBALLS

Phase 2 *Elimination*

Low FODMAP

If you are craving something sweet and need a treat, try making this recipe! The coconut fat will help you feel satiated when on a restricted diet. Try substituting organic peppermint extract or organic orange flavoring (after you have introduced and tested okay for citrus) for the vanilla powder.

⅔ cup coconut butter

3 tablespoons virgin coconut oil

1 tablespoon raw honey (optional)

1 cup unsweetened shredded coconut, plus extra for rolling

½ teaspoon raw vanilla powder

pinch sea salt

Place the coconut butter and coconut oil in a small saucepan and warm over the lowest heat until softened but not completely melted. Pour the mixture into a food processor fitted with the "s" blade. Add the honey and process for a few seconds. Then add the shredded coconut, vanilla powder, and salt. Process until combined.

Scoop the mixture into a bowl and form it into balls. If the mixture is too soft to form, place the bowl in the refrigerator for about 30 minutes, then try again. Roll each ball in shredded coconut and serve. Store extra snowballs in an airtight container in the refrigerator for up to a month.

Yield: about 12 snowballs

TIP

To measure coconut butter from the jar, first make sure it is at room temperature, then take a butter knife and cut it up into little chunks in the jar. Then pour the little chunks into a measuring cup.

CHAI-SPICED SUNFLOWER TRUFFLES

Phase 2 *Elimination*

Having a recipe like this made up in your refrigerator will be extremely helpful during the strict part of the Elimination Diet—phase 2. Otherwise you may get tempted to grab anything when hungry. Make up a big batch of this recipe and store it in a covered glass container for up to two weeks!

2 cups raw sunflower seeds
1 tablespoon ground cinnamon
1 teaspoon ground ginger
½ teaspoon ground cardamom
pinch sea salt

1 cup pitted Medjool dates
2 tablespoons extra-virgin olive oil
1 to 2 tablespoons pure maple syrup
   or raw honey (optional)
unsweetened shredded coconut

Place the sunflower seeds, spices, and salt in a food processor fitted with the "s" blade. Process until the seeds are very finely ground. It only takes a minute or so.

Add the pitted dates and oil. Process again until combined and sticky. Check to see if you can form a truffle by rolling some of the mixture in your hands. If it falls apart, then add the maple syrup and process again.

Scoop out the sunflower mixture by the large spoonful and roll it into balls. Roll the balls in shredded coconut. Store leftover truffles in an airtight container in the refrigerator for up to 2 weeks.

Yield: about 24 truffles

PUMPKIN SEED BUTTER ENERGY BARS

Phase 2 *Elimination*

Keep these bars in your freezer for the times when you are feeling very hungry and in need of a nutrient-dense snack immediately. We use Omega Nutrition pumpkin seed butter. Look for it at your local health food store or order it online.

¾ cup pitted Medjool dates (about 8)

½ cup shredded unsweetened coconut

¼ cup dried currants or raisins

1 to 2 teaspoons ground cinnamon

¼ teaspoon raw vanilla powder

¾ cup pumpkin seed butter

⅓ cup melted coconut butter

Line a 9 x 5-inch glass bread pan with unbleached parchment paper.

Place the dates, shredded coconut, currants, cinnamon, and vanilla powder in a food processor fitted with the "s" blade. Process the mixture for about 30 seconds, and then add the remaining ingredients. Process again until combined.

Pour the mixture into the prepared bread pan. Place it in your freezer for about 1 hour to set. Then cut into bars with a very sharp knife. Serve. Keep any leftover bars in the freezer until ready to serve—they will become soft at room temperature.

Yield: about 10 bars

TIP

To melt coconut butter, place a few large spoonfuls in a small saucepan and melt on the stovetop over the lowest heat, then measure out ⅓ cup.

AVOCADO-MINT MINI TARTS

Phase 3 *Reintroduction (citrus)*

Use this recipe when challenging citrus in phase 3. This recipe is so simple to make and yet looks like a gourmet masterpiece when all is said and done. I use a muffin tin lined with unbleached paper muffin cups for my "tart" pan. First, you press the crust mixture into the bottom of each muffin cup, then you add the filling. Then the whole muffin tin is placed in the freezer to "set" the tarts. You can take one out at a time and enjoy them slowly or bring the whole pan out to share with guests.

CRUST

1½ cups shredded unsweetened coconut

½ cup hemp seeds

¼ teaspoon raw vanilla powder (optional)

pinch sea salt

6 soft Medjool dates, pitted

2 to 3 teaspoons coconut oil

FILLING

4 small ripe avocados

6 tablespoons melted coconut oil

6 tablespoons freshly squeezed lime juice

4 tablespoons raw honey

1 handful fresh mint leaves

Line a 12-cup muffin pan with unbleached paper liners.

To make the crust, place the shredded coconut, hemp seeds, vanilla powder, and salt in a food processor fitted with the "s" blade and process until finely ground. Add the dates and oil; continue processing until the mixture comes together. Divide the crust mixture evenly among the prepared muffin cups and press it firmly into the bottom of each.

To make the filling, place all the ingredients for the filling in a food processor fitted with the "s" blade and process until smooth and creamy. Pour or scoop the mixture into the muffin cups over the crust, dividing it evenly.

Freeze the muffin pan for 1 to 2 hours or until the tart filling is firm to the touch. When ready to serve, remove the tarts from the pan and then remove the paper liners before serving.

Yield: 12 mini tarts

ALMOND BUTTER COOKIES

Phase 3 *Reintroduction (almonds)*

Make this recipe during phase 3 when you are testing almonds. I like to serve them with homemade Raw Vanilla Almond Milk (page 290). They are crispy on the outside and chewy in the center. To grind chia seeds, place at least ¼ cup in a coffee grinder or Vitamix and grind. Store any leftovers in a glass jar in the fridge.

WET INGREDIENTS	DRY INGREDIENTS
2 tablespoons ground chia seeds	1½ cups brown rice flour
¼ cup warm water	½ teaspoon sea salt
¼ cup unsweetened applesauce	½ teaspoon baking soda
¼ cup softened coconut oil	
¾ cup coconut sugar	
1 cup roasted almond butter	

Preheat the oven to 350°F.

Place the ground chia seeds and warm water into a medium mixing bowl; whisk together. Then add the remaining wet ingredients. Beat together with an electric mixer or vigorously mix together with a wooden spoon.

In a separate bowl, whisk together the dry ingredients. Add the dry ingredients to the bowl with the wet and beat again until the dough forms a ball. The dough will be sticky and may ride up on the beaters. If this happens, just turn the mixer off and scrape off the dough, then mix again.

Roll the dough into balls, place them on a cookie sheet, and press down using the tines of a fork. Bake for 10 to 12 minutes. Cool on a wire rack.

Yield: about twenty-four 2-inch cookies

CHOCOLATE ZUCCHINI CUPCAKES

Phase 3 *Reintroduction (chocolate)*

Use this recipe when challenging chocolate in phase 3. I know, the Elimination Diet is so rough! Serve with a dollop of Whipped Vanilla Coconut Cream (page 280) on top of each cupcake for a decadent treat.

DRY INGREDIENTS

1 cup brown rice flour

½ cup arrowroot powder or tapioca flour

¼ cup raw cacao powder

1 teaspoon baking soda

¼ teaspoon sea salt

WET INGREDIENTS

2 tablespoons ground chia seeds

¼ cup warm water

¾ cup unsweetened applesauce

¾ cup coconut sugar

½ cup melted coconut oil, plus more for greasing the pan

2 teaspoons raw apple cider vinegar

1½ cups grated raw zucchini

Preheat the oven to 350°F. Grease a 12-cup muffin pan with coconut oil or line the wells with unbleached paper liners.

In a medium mixing bowl, whisk together the dry ingredients. In a separate mixing bowl, vigorously whisk together the ground chia seeds and warm water. Add the applesauce, sugar, coconut oil, and vinegar; beat together. Stir in the zucchini.

Pour the wet ingredients into the dry and stir together with a large wooden spoon until combined. Scoop the batter into the prepared muffin cups, filling them about halfway full.

Bake for 20 to 25 minutes. Cool on a wire rack. Serve.

Yield: 12 cupcakes

PUMPKIN PIE CHIA PUDDING

Phase 3 *Reintroduction (cashews)*

This recipe is a delicious way to challenge cashews in phase 3, or try the following variation using coconut milk and enjoy this dessert during phase 2. This raw pudding is similar to tapioca pudding. The chia seeds expand and release their gelatinous substance when soaked in a liquid. Serve pudding in small bowls topped with Whipped Vanilla Coconut Cream (page 280) and freshly grated nutmeg. If you do not own a high-powered blender, you will want to soak the cashews for about 3 hours before blending them.

½ cup raw cashews

1½ cups water

½ cup pure pumpkin purée

4 to 6 tablespoons pure maple syrup or coconut nectar

2 teaspoons pumpkin pie spice

pinch sea salt

6 tablespoons whole chia seeds

Place the cashews, water, pumpkin purée, maple syrup, pie spice, and salt in a high-powered blender and blend until smooth and ultra-creamy. Pour into a medium bowl or glass container.

Add the chia seeds and whisk together. Let soak at room temperature for about 1 hour. Then cover and transfer to the refrigerator to soak and thicken for at least 2 more hours, or preferably overnight.

Scoop into small bowls and serve.

Yield: about 6 servings

TIP

Use white chia seeds for a lighter-colored pudding or use the black variety for a darker-colored pudding.

Phase 2 VARIATION

Replace the raw cashews and water with 1 (14.5-ounce) can full-fat organic coconut milk for a nut-free version.

PEACHY COCONUT CREAMSICLES

Phase 2 *Elimination*

Having healthy treats on hand is so helpful to succeeding on the Elimination Diet, especially if your child is participating in it. Look for stainless steel Popsicle molds. See the Resources section on page 303 for more information.

2 ripe medium peaches

½ small avocado

2 to 3 soft Medjool dates, pitted

1 (14.5-ounce) can coconut milk

¼ to ½ teaspoon raw vanilla powder (optional)

Place all the ingredients in a high-powered blender and blend until smooth and creamy. Pour into Popsicle molds and freeze until firm, 3 to 6 hours. When ready to serve, run the mold under hot running water to release the creamsicles from the mold.

Yield: 8 to 10 creamsicles, depending on the size of your molds

---

TIP

Use 2 cups frozen peach slices if fresh peaches are out of season. Also, if your dates are rather hard and dry, soak them for 30 minutes in warm water before using them in this recipe.

CUCUMBER-MINT WATER

Phase 1 *Detox*

Low FODMAP

Drinking water is so vitally important to detoxing. This infused water makes drinking lots of water more enjoyable! Always make sure you are drinking, and cooking with, filtered water, as chemicals and drug residues in city water can wreak havoc on your health. For one thing, these chemicals kill off friendly bacteria in the gut, and two, the drug residues can affect your hormone balance, possibly causing unexplained weight gain. If you don't have a reverse osmosis water filtration system installed in your kitchen, then buy 5-gallon jugs of filtered water from your local health food store at a refillable water station.

---

7 cups filtered water   4 to 6 sprigs fresh mint
1 small cucumber, cut into thin slices

Pour 3½ cups filtered water into each of two quart jars. Evenly distribute the cucumber slices and fresh mint between the two jars. Cover each jar with a lid. Let them sit on your counter for 2 hours, then transfer to the refrigerator. Sip the water throughout the day.

Yield: 2 quarts

RAW VANILLA ALMOND MILK

Phase 3 *Reintroduction (almonds)*

Use raw almond milk as a base for creamy fruit smoothies, in baked goods in place of dairy milk, or top warm whole-grain breakfast cereals. I also like to add it to warm spice tea or just drink it plain—it's so delicious!

1 cup raw almonds	½ teaspoon raw vanilla powder
4 cups water	pinch sea salt
1 tablespoon pure maple syrup	

Place the almonds in a small bowl and cover with filtered water. Soak at room temperature for 8 to 12 hours, or overnight.

After the almonds have soaked, drain them and rinse them well under warm running water. Place them in a blender with the 4 cups water, maple syrup, vanilla, and salt and blend on high for 1 to 2 minutes, or until you have a very smooth milk.

Pour the milk through a fine-mesh strainer lined with cheesecloth, or a nut milk bag, into a container and squeeze out as much milk from the pulp as possible.

Store in a covered glass jar in the refrigerator for up to 3 days.

Yield: about 4 cups

VANILLA HEMP MILK

Phase 2 *Elimination*

Low FODMAP

Use hemp milk to top hot whole-grain breakfast cereals, as a base for smoothies, or as a refreshing drink. It can also be used in baking recipes where milk is called for. Hemp milk takes just minutes to make.

½ cup shelled hemp seeds	½ teaspoon raw vanilla powder
3 cups filtered water	pinch sea salt
1 tablespoon maple syrup	

Place all the ingredients in a high-powered blender and blend for 60 to 90 seconds, or until ultra-smooth. Use as is, or strain it for a smoother consistency. To strain, place a nut milk bag in a large jar or pitcher and pour the hemp milk through the bag, squeezing out the milk and leaving the pulp behind.

Store your hemp milk in a tightly covered glass jar in the refrigerator for 3 to 4 days.

Yield: about 3 cups

VANILLA CASHEW MILK

Phase 3 *Reintroduction (cashews)*

Use this recipe when you are challenging cashews during phase 3. If you don't have a reaction, then continue using this recipe throughout the rest of the diet. It's delicious drizzled over warm whole-grain breakfast cereals, added to warm spice tea in place of cow's milk, or enjoyed as a creamy beverage.

½ cup raw cashews	¼ teaspoon raw vanilla powder
3 cups water	pinch sea salt
2 to 3 teaspoons raw honey or pure maple syrup	

Place all the ingredients in a high-powered blender and blend until ultra-smooth and creamy. Add more water for a thinner consistency.

Yield: 3½ cups

WARMING SPICE TEA

`Phase 1` *Detox*

This tea has a warming flavor that's similar to chai tea, but without the black tea (which contains caffeine). Drink this digestive-supportive tea any time of day—it's especially good after a meal. Once you are in phase 2, you can add Vanilla Hemp Milk (page 290), or for phase 3, try adding Raw Vanilla Almond Milk (page 290). Add a little honey to sweeten it, if desired.

4 cups water

2 cinnamon sticks, broken into pieces

5 to 6 cardamom pods, crushed

1 teaspoon whole cloves

1 teaspoon whole black peppercorns

2 tablespoons thinly sliced fresh ginger

milk of your choice

raw honey

Place the water and spices in a 2-quart pot. Cover the pot with a lid, bring to a gentle boil, then reduce the heat and simmer for 10 to 15 minutes. Strain the tea through a fine-mesh strainer into a quart jar. Pour into mugs, top off with the milk of your choice (if you are in phase 2 or 3), and sweeten to taste with raw honey.

Yield: 4 cups

`Phase 3` **VARIATION**

Add raw organic cream or whole milk to this tea when challenging dairy in the last stages of phase 3.

NIGHTTIME TEA

Phase 1 *Detox*

Low FODMAP

Sleeping well is key to proper digestion and detoxification. When we don't sleep, our bodies produce more inflammatory chemicals. This can lead to a leaky gut, as well as pain and inflammation throughout the body. This tea calms the nervous system and helps prepare the body for a deep sleep. Drink 1 to 2 cups about one hour before bedtime.

1 tablespoon dried chamomile
1 tablespoon dried passionflower
1 tablespoon dried catnip

1 tablespoon dried spearmint
1 tablespoon dried rosebuds
6 cups boiling water

Place the herbs in an 8-cup glass liquid measuring cup. Pour the boiling water over them, cover with a plate, and let steep for 5 to 7 minutes.

Strain the tea, discarding the solids, and drink. Store any leftover tea in a glass jar in the refrigerator, then reheat in a small pot as needed.

Yield: 6 cups

TIP

Make sure you purchase organic rosebuds. If you can't find organic, just omit them from the recipe. Conventional rose farming is very chemical-intensive. These chemicals can change the way our bodies respond to food, as well as alter the bacteria in our guts.

ADRENAL SUPPORT TEA

Phase 1 *Detox*

Low FODMAP

The majority of people are walking around under constant stress. This can change digestion and immune system functions and leave you more susceptible to having a leaky gut. Science is even showing that stress can alter the organisms in our intestinal tract. This tea contains herbs that have been shown to assist in normalizing the stress response.

---

4 cups water	2 tablespoons dried ashwagandha
2 tablespoons dried licorice root	2 tablespoons sliced fresh ginger

---

Place all the ingredients in a 2-quart pot. Cover the pot with a lid, bring to a gentle boil, then reduce the heat and simmer for 15 to 20 minutes.

Strain the tea, discarding the solids in the strainer, and drink. If the tea is too strong for you, add more hot water to your mug to dilute it. Store any leftover tea in a glass jar in the refrigerator, then reheat in a small pot as needed.

Yield: 4 cups

CHICKEN STOCK

Phase 1 *Detox*

Chicken stock can be used during all phases of the diet. It's rich in gut-healing nutrients, amino acids, minerals, and vitamins. Chicken stock can be made two different ways—from a chicken carcass that has been previously roasted or from a fresh, whole chicken. If you use a fresh, whole chicken, cook the stock for no more than 2 hours. This option produces a lot of cooked meat that can be stored in your refrigerator, which can be used to make a quick Elimination Diet meal.

bones and skin from 2 roasted organic chickens (meat picked off)
1 pound fresh chicken wings
1 large onion, chopped
1 head garlic, cut in half crosswise
4 celery stalks, chopped
2 carrots, chopped
3 to 4 sprigs fresh thyme
2 to 3 sprigs fresh rosemary
1 handful fresh parsley
1 to 2 teaspoons whole black peppercorns
2 bay leaves
2 teaspoons sea salt
16 cups filtered water
1 tablespoon raw apple cider vinegar

Place all the ingredients in an 8-quart stockpot, cover, and bring to a gentle boil, then reduce the heat to low and simmer for 6 to 8 hours. Strain the stock through a large stainless steel colander into a large bowl or another 8-quart pot. Discard the solids in the strainer.

Pour the stock into quart jars, cover, and refrigerate for up to 5 days, or freeze for longer storage.

Yield: about 3 quarts

VEGETABLE-SEAWEED STOCK

Phase 1 *Detox*

Stocks are actually very easy to prepare. You just toss everything into a big pot, cover, and let it simmer for hours on your stove. If you don't have all of the ingredients, don't worry—stocks are very forgiving, so just use the ingredients that you have on hand. The seaweeds add an abundance of trace minerals to the stock, which is very beneficial as most people are deficient in minerals. Freeze your stock in widemouthed quart jars for later use.

1 large onion, coarsely chopped	2 tablespoons arame or hijiki
1 leek, rinsed and chopped	1 tablespoon dulse flakes
2 to 3 carrots, chopped	1 sprig fresh rosemary
4 celery stalks, chopped	1 sprig fresh thyme
4 garlic cloves, chopped	3 bay leaves
½ bunch fresh parsley	1 teaspoon whole black peppercorns
2 strips kombu	16 cups filtered water

Place all the ingredients in an 8-quart stockpot and bring to a boil. Cover, reduce the heat to low, and simmer for 3 to 4 hours.

Strain the stock through a large stainless steel colander into another pot, discard the vegetables, and pour the stock into clean, widemouthed 1-quart jars. Store the stock in the refrigerator for up to a week, or freeze for longer storage.

Yield: 4 quarts

PICKLED CAULIFLOWER, CARROTS, AND GREEN BEANS

Phase 2 *Elimination*

Fermentation is a magical process where beneficial bacteria present on vegetables are allowed to flourish under the right conditions—an anaerobic environment made possible by a salt brine and a covered jar. Lacto-fermented vegetables are rich sources of probiotics that your digestive system needs to thrive! Eat a few tablespoons of these vegetables with every meal.

LEARN MORE ABOUT FERMENTED FOODS

For more delicious fermented vegetable recipes, check out *The Whole Life Nutrition Cookbook*. There you will find an entire chapter dedicated to cultured and fermented foods, including dairy-free yogurt, kombucha, coconut water kefir, dilly carrots and green beans, zucchini dill kraut, pickled basil beets, and many more. Also be sure to visit our recipe blog, NourishingMeals.com, where you will find a video on how to make lacto-fermented vegetables—videos make learning new things so much easier!

---

2 to 3 sprigs fresh dill
1 teaspoon whole black peppercorns
2 cups chopped cauliflower
1 cup chopped green beans

1 cup diced carrots
2 cups filtered water
1 to 1½ tablespoons sea salt
1 large cabbage leaf

Place the dill and black peppercorns in the bottom of a glass quart jar. Layer the cauliflower, green beans, and carrots on top of them. Pack them in tightly.

Whisk together the water and salt in a small bowl or 2-cup glass liquid measuring cup. Make sure the salt has dissolved, and then pour the mixture over the vegetables until they are covered with at least ½ inch of brine. Fold the cabbage leaf up and press it into the vegetables to ensure that they stay below the brine. Cover tightly with a plastic lid and place in an undisturbed spot in your kitchen away from direct sunlight for 5 to 7 days, or until soured to your liking.

When you begin to see a lot of bubbling, after day 2 to 3, gently unscrew the lid to release excess gases, then screw it back down tightly. This is called "burping" the jar. Do this 1 to 2 times a day until the vegetables have fermented (soured) to your liking.

Store your pickled vegetables in the refrigerator for 3 to 6 months.

Yield: 1 quart

VARIATIONS

Nearly any diced raw vegetable will work in this recipe. Try red radishes, daikon radish, red onions, turnips, garlic cloves, garlic scapes, or red bell peppers and hot chiles (only during phase 3).

TIP

Make sure you chop the vegetables into small pieces—this will help them to ferment properly.

DILL PICKLED TURNIPS

Phase 2 *Elimination*

Low FODMAP

Turnips come in various sizes—from small, radish-size ones to large enough to fill up the palm of your hand. Use about two bunches of small or about two larger ones. This low-FODMAP recipe is delicious served with breakfast, lunch, or dinner!

½ bunch fresh dill	2 cups filtered water
½ bunch green onions, chopped	1 to 1½ tablespoons sea salt
3½ cups chopped turnips	1 large cabbage leaf

Place the dill and chopped green onions in the bottom of a glass quart jar. Add the chopped turnips to fill the jar to about 2 inches below the top. Pack them in tightly.

Whisk together the water and salt in a small bowl or 2-cup glass liquid measuring cup. Make sure the salt has dissolved, and then pour the mixture over the vegetables until they are covered with at least ½ inch of brine. Fold the cabbage leaf up and press it into the vegetables to ensure that they stay below the brine. Cover tightly with a plastic lid and place in an undisturbed spot in your kitchen away from direct sunlight for 5 to 7 days, or until soured to your liking.

When you begin to see a lot of bubbling, after day 2 to 3, gently unscrew the lid to release excess gases, then screw it back down tightly. This is called "burping" the jar. Do this 1 to 2 times a day until the vegetables have fermented (soured) to your liking.

Store your pickled vegetables in the refrigerator for 3 to 6 months.

Yield: 1 quart

RAINBOW KRAUT

Phase 2 *Elimination*

Low FODMAP

This recipe gets its name because of the red cabbage, green cabbage, and carrots used. Start a batch of the sauerkraut about one week before you begin the Elimination Diet. This way it will be ready for you when you enter phase 2. Serve a few spoonfuls of this kraut with every meal.

4 cups thinly sliced red cabbage (about ¾ pound)	2 large carrots, grated
4 cups thinly sliced green cabbage (about ¾ pound)	1 tablespoon sea salt
	1 large cabbage leaf

Place all of the ingredients, except the whole cabbage leaf, in a large bowl and pound with a wooden kraut pounder or another blunt object until the juices from the vegetables are released. This usually takes 5 to 10 minutes of continuous pounding.

Spoon the kraut into a glass quart jar, packing the kraut in tight by pressing down with the kraut pounder until the juices rise above the vegetables. Make sure to leave about 1 inch of space from the top of the jar. Fold up the cabbage leaf and press it into the juices so they at least partially rise above it. Screw a plastic lid on tightly.

Place the jar into another container or baking dish to catch any leaking juices, then place in a spot in your house away from direct sunlight. Let the kraut ferment for 5 to 10 days. Fermentation will take place faster in warmer weather and slower in cooler weather.

When you begin to see a lot of bubbling, after day 2 to 3, gently unscrew the lid to release excess gases, then screw it back down tightly. This is called "burping" the jar. Do this 1 to 2 times a day until the vegetables have fermented (soured) to your liking. If your kraut has lost a bit of brine from leakage, then replace what was lost with extra brine. Use 1 cup filtered water mixed with 1½ teaspoons sea salt. Then add this mixture to the kraut until it is about ½ inch from the top of the jar. Screw the lid back on tightly and let it continue to ferment. Taste your kraut after about 5 days. If it is sour and tangy, then it is done; if not, let it continue to ferment.

Store your kraut in the refrigerator for 3 to 6 months.

Yield: 1 quart

FRESH BROCCOLI SPROUTS

Phase 2 *Elimination*

Low FODMAP

Growing your own little sprout garden is a fun and exciting process. Broccoli seeds are particularly challenging to sprout, as they take longer to sprout compared to other seeds, so be patient. It takes a few days for the seeds to even break open, and they are slow in growing. They say that all good things come to those who wait. Broccoli sprouts are very good things, so your patience will be rightfully rewarded (see page 105 for the benefits of these sprouts).

TIP

Broccoli sprouts have a spicy flavor and are not tolerated by some. You may want to mix the broccoli seeds with radish, clover, or alfalfa seeds for a different flavor before sprouting.

---

2 tablespoons sprouting seeds
(organic broccoli seeds)

Place the seeds into a widemouthed quart jar with a spouting lid and cover them with a few inches of warm purified water. Let them soak overnight in a warm dark place. After 8 to 10 hours, drain off the water.

Rinse the seeds with fresh water, 3 to 4 times a day for 4 to 5 days. Place the jar in a warm, dark place during this time period. Make sure to drain off all of the water after each rinsing to prevent spoiling of the sprouts. (I know you are excited to grow your own garden right in your kitchen, but it will likely take 2 to 3 days for the seeds to split open and have the sprouts show, so be patient.)

Once your sprouts are a few centimeters long and have defined yellow leaves, move your jar out to a place where it can be exposed to some sunlight.

This will allow the sprouts to harvest sunlight and grow quickly. Be sure to keep rinsing them, as the sprouts can dry out quickly in hot and dry environments. You will recognize when the sprouts are ready as they will have darker green leaves and be about an inch or longer in length. Don't worry about eating them too early. As soon as they are green, they are ready to go.

Yield: about 4 cups

TIP

See our video and other information about sprouting on our website at WholeLifeNutrition.net.

RESOURCES

Oils and Vinegars

Organic Virgin Coconut Oil: www.TropicalTraditions.com; www.Nutiva.com

Organic Extra-Virgin Olive Oil: www.Bionaturae.com

Raw Apple Cider Vinegar: www.Bragg.com

Raw Coconut Vinegar: www.CoconutSecret.com

Organic Raw Nuts and Seeds

Chia and Hemp Seeds: www.Nutiva.com

Pumpkin and Sunflower Seeds: www.LivingTreeCommunity.com

Unpasteurized Organic Raw Almonds: www.organicalmondsraw.com

Nut and Seed Butters

Raw Cashew Butter: www.ArtisanaFoods.com

Roasted Almond Butter: www.ZinkeOrchards.com

Pumpkin Seed Butter: www.OmegaNutrition.com

Organic Meats and Wild Seafood

Pasture Raised Organic Meats: www.UsWellnessMeats.com; www.TropicalTraditions.com

Wild Seafood: www.VitalChoice.com

Organic Whole Grains and Noodles

Brown and White Rice: www.BobsRedMill.com

Sprouted Brown Rice: www.PlanetRiceFoods.com

Quinoa: www.BobsRedMill.com; www.Quinoa.net (Ancient Harvest)

Sprouted Quinoa: www.TruRoots.com

Quinoa-rice Noodles: www.AndeanDream.com

Brown Rice Noodles: www.Tinkyada.com

Gluten-Free Flours

Blanched Almond Flour: www.Nuts.com; www.LucysKitchenShop.com

Arrowroot Powder: www.BobsRedMill.com

Coconut Flour: www.BobsRedMill.com; www.TropicalTraditions.com;
www.Nutiva.com

Sprouted Brown Rice Flour: www.PlanetRiceFoods.com;
www.OrganicSproutedFlour.net

Sprouted Garbanzo Bean Flour: www.OrganicSproutedFlour.net

Quinoa Flour: www.BobsRedMill.com; www.Quinoa.net (Ancient Harvest)

Other Ingredients

Organic Raw Vanilla Powder: www.DivineOrganics.com

Raw Organic Cacao Powder: www.EssentialLivingFoods.com;
www.NavitasNaturals.com

Maca Powder: www.EssentialLivingFoods.com;
www.NavitasNaturals.com

Supplements

After working as a medical affairs member for Thorne Research for seven years, I learned that all supplement products are not created equal. Many suppliers are cutting their costs by purchasing substandard raw materials that may be contaminated with harmful microbes or toxic chemicals. It is of utmost importance that you buy supplements from a reputable company. While there are many good companies out there, I have listed the particular products below because I have had outstanding success with them in clinical practice. Visit the Supplement section of our website, WholeLife Nutrition.net.

Multivitamin: Thorne Research Basic Nutrients 2/day, www.Thorne.com

Vitamin D: www.GrassrootsHealth.com; Thorne Research Vitamin D/K2 Liquid, www.Thorne.com

Essential Fatty Acids: www.NordicNaturals.com

Magnesium Citrate: Thorne Research Magnesium Citrate, www.Thorne .com

Activated Charcoal: www.SwansonVitamins.com

Amino Acids

If you would like a custom blend of amino acids made to match your specific needs, you can visit this link for further details on lab testing and custom formulas: www.metabolicmaintenance.com/amino-acid-formulas

Broad Spectrum: Thorne Amino Acid Complex, www.Thorne.com

L-Glutamine: Thorne L-Glutamine Powder, www.Thorne.com

N-Acetyl Cysteine: Thorne Cysteplus, www.Thorne.com

Solvent Remover: www.Thorne.com

Probiotics: www.Klaire.com; www.BodyBiotics.com; www.Culturelle.com; www.Florastor.com; www.PhillipsRelief.com; www.SwansonVitamins.com

Berberine: Thorne Berberine-500, www.Thorne.com

Meriva: Thorne Meriva-500, www.Thorne.com

Betaine HCL with Pepsin: www.Thorne.com

Digestive Enzymes: Bio-Gest, www.Thorne.com; Digest Gold, www.Enzymedica-Digest.com

Kitchen Equipment

High-Powered Blender: www.Vitamix.com; www.Blendtec.com

Stainless Steel Immersion Blender: www.Cuisinart.com

Food Processor: www.Cuisinart.com

Stainless Steel Popsicle Molds: www.OnyxContainers.com

Stainless Steel Food Storage Containers: www.LifeWithoutPlastic.com

Stone Bakeware: www.PamperedChef.com

Books and Websites

Rich Food, Poor Food: The Ultimate Grocery Purchasing System by Jason and Mira Calton

The Institute for Functional Medicine: www.functionalmedicine.org

Finding a Functional Medicine Practitioner: www.functionalmedicine.org/Patients/Resources/#FAP

The Feingold Diet, phenol/salicylate-free diet: www.Feingold.org

REFERENCES

Chapter 1

Hicklin JA, McEwen LM, Morgan JE. The effect of diet in rheumatoid arthritis. *Clin Allergy.* 1980; 10: 463.

Grant EC. Food allergies and migraine. *Lancet.* 1979 May 5; 1(8123): 966–9.

Breneman JC. Allergy elimination diet as the most effective gallbladder diet. *Ann Allergy.* 1968; 26: 83–7.

Ruuskanen A, Kaukinen K, Collin P, Huhtala H, Valve R, Maki M, et al. Positive serum antigliadin antibodies without celiac disease in the elderly population: does it matter? *Scand J Gastroenterol.* 2010; 45: 1197–202.

Jackson KD, Howie LD, Akinbami LJ. Trends in allergic conditions among children: United States, 1997–2011. Food allergies increased 50%. *NCHS Data Brief.* 2013 May; (121): 1–8.

Sicherer SH, Muñoz-Furlong A, Godbold JH, et al. US prevalence of self-reported peanut, tree nut, and sesame allergy: 11-year follow-up. *J Allergy Clin Immunol.* 2010 Jun; 125(6): 1322–6

www.webmd.com/allergies/allergy-statistics.

Pribila BA, Hertzler SR, Martin BR, et al. Improved lactose digestion and intolerance among African-American adolescent girls fed a dairy-rich diet. *J Am Diet Assoc.* 2000 May; 100(5): 524–8; quiz 529–30.

Wood RA, Segall N, Ahlstedt S, et al. Accuracy of IgE antibody laboratory results. *Ann Allergy Asthma Immunol.* 2007 Jul; 99(1): 34–41.

Lavine E. Blood testing for sensitivity, allergy or intolerance to food. *CMAJ.* cmaj.110026; published ahead of print March 19, 2012, doi: 10.1503/cmaj.110026.

Wilders-Truschnig M, Mangge H, Lieners C, et al. IgG antibodies against food antigens are correlated with inflammation and intima media thickness in obese juveniles. *Exp Clin Endocrinol Diabetes.* 2008 Apr; 116(4): 241–5.

Chapter 2

Cassady BA, Hollis JH, Fulford AD, et al. Mastication of almonds: effects of lipid bioaccessibility, appetite, and hormone response. *Am J Clin Nutr*. 2009 Mar; 89(3): 794–800. PMID: 19144727.

Mansueto P, Montalto G, Pacor ML, et al. Food allergy in gastroenterologic diseases: review of literature. *World J Gastroenterol*. 2006 Dec 28; 12(48): 7744–52.

Untersmayr E, Bakos N, Schöll I, et al. Anti-ulcer drugs promote IgE formation toward dietary antigens in adult patients. *FASEB J*. 2005 Apr; 19(6): 656–8.

Prichard PJ, Yeomans ND, Mihaly GW, et al. Omeprazole: a study of its inhibition of gastric pH and oral pharmacokinetics after morning or evening dosage. *Gastroenterology*. 1985 Jan; 88(1 Pt 1): 64–9.

Heidelbaugh JJ, Goldberg KL, Inadomi JM. Overutilization of proton pump inhibitors: a review of cost-effectiveness and risk [corrected]. *Am J Gastroenterol*. 2009 Mar; 104 Suppl 2: S27–32.

Riemer AB, Gruber S, Pali-Schöll I, et al. Suppression of gastric acid increases the risk of developing immunoglobulin E-mediated drug hypersensitivity: human diclofenac sensitization and a murine sensitization model. *Clin Exp Allergy*. 2010 Mar; 40(3): 486–93.

Moreno FJ. Gastrointestinal digestion of food allergens: effect on their allergenicity. *Biomed Pharmacother*. Jan 2007; 61(1): 50–60.

Breneman JC. Allergy elimination diet as the most effective gallbladder diet. *Ann Allergy*. 1968; 26: 83–7.

Malterre T. Digestive and nutritional considerations in celiac disease: could supplementation help? *Altern Med Rev*. 2009 Sep; 14(3): 247–57.

Leeds JS, Hopper AD, Hurlstone DP, et al. Is exocrine pancreatic insufficiency in adult coeliac disease a cause of persisting symptoms? *Aliment Pharmacol Ther*. 2007 Feb 1; 25(3): 265–71.

Damm I, Mikkat U, Kirchhoff F, et al. Inhibitory effect of the lectin wheat germ agglutinin on the binding of 125I-CCK-8s to the CCK-A and -B receptors of AR42J cells. *Pancreas*. 2004 Jan; 28(1): 31–7.

Rossi M, Amaretti A, Raimondi S. Folate production by probiotic bacteria. *Nutrients*. 2011 January; 3(1): 118–34.

Pompei A, Cordisco L, Amaretti A, et al. Folate production by bifidobacteria as a potential probiotic property. *Appl Environ Microbiol*. 2007 Jan; 73(1): 179–85.

LeBlanc JG, Laiño JE, del Valle MJ, et al. B-group vitamin production by lactic acid bacteria—current knowledge and potential applications. *J Appl Microbiol*. 2011 Dec; 111(6): 1297–309.

Madara J. Building an intestine—architectural contributions of commensal bacteria. *N Engl J Med*. 2004 Oct 14; 351(16): 1685–6.

Petrof EO, Claud EC, Gloor GB, et al. Microbial ecosystems therapeutics: a new paradigm in medicine? *Benef Microbes*. 2013 Mar 1; 4(1): 53–65.

Norman JM, Handley SA, Virgin HW. Kingdom-agnostic metagenomics and the importance of complete characterization of enteric microbial communities. *Gastroenterology*. 2014 May; 146(6): 1459–69.

Sleator RD. The human superorganism—of microbes and men. *Med Hypotheses*. 2010 Feb; 74(2): 214–5.

David LA, Maurice CF, Carmody RN, et al. Diet rapidly and reproducibly alters the human gut microbiome. *Nature*. 2014 Jan 23; 505(7484): 559–63.

Ménard S, Cerf-Bensussan N, Heyman M. Multiple facets of intestinal permeability and epithelial handling of dietary antigens. *Mucosal Immunol*. 2010 May; 3(3): 247–59.

Horton F, Wright J, Smith L, et al. Increased intestinal permeability to oral chromium (51 Cr) -EDTA in human Type 2 diabetes. *Diabet Med*. 2014 May; 31(5): 559–63.

Visser J, Rozing J, Sapone A, et al. Tight junctions, intestinal permeability, and autoimmunity: celiac disease and type 1 diabetes paradigms. *Ann N Y Acad Sci*. 2009 May; 1165: 195–205.

Fasano A. Leaky gut and autoimmune diseases. *Clin Rev Allergy Immunol*. 2012 Feb; 42(1): 71–8.

Fasano A. Zonulin, regulation of tight junctions, and autoimmune diseases. *Ann N Y Acad Sci*. 2012 Jul; 1258: 25–33.

Von Geldern G, Mowry EM. The influence of nutritional factors on the prognosis of multiple sclerosis. *Nat Rev Neurol*. 2012 Dec; 8(12): 678–89.

Chapter 3

Drago S, El Asmar R, Di Pierro M, et al. Gliadin, zonulin and gut permeability: effects on celiac and non-celiac intestinal mucosa and intestinal cell lines. *Scand J Gastroenterol*. 2006 Apr; 41(4): 408–19.

Damm I, Mikkat U, Kirchhoff F, et al. Inhibitory effect of the lectin wheat germ agglutinin on the binding of 125I-CCK-8s to the CCK-A and -B receptors of AR42J cells. *Pancreas*. 2004 Jan; 28(1): 31–7.

Lebwohl B, Blaser MJ, Ludvigsson JF, et al. Decreased risk of celiac disease in patients with *Helicobacter pylori* colonization. *Am J Epidemiol*. 2013 Dec 15; 178(12): 1721–30.

D'Arienzo R, Maurano F, Luongo D, et al. Adjuvant effect of *Lactobacillus casei* in a mouse model of gluten sensitivity. *Immunol Lett*. 2008 Aug 15; 119(1–2): 78–83.

Pozo-Rubio T, Olivares M, Nova E, et al. Immune development and intestinal microbiota in celiac disease. *Clin Dev Immunol*. 2012; article ID 654143, 12 pages.

Sellitto M, Bai G, Serena G, et al. Proof of concept of microbiome-metabolome analysis and delayed gluten exposure on celiac disease autoimmunity in genetically at-risk infants. *PLoS One*. 2012; 7(3): e33387.

Cotter PD, Stanton C, Ross RP, et al. The impact of antibiotics on the gut microbiota as revealed by high throughput DNA sequencing. *Discov Med*. 2012 Mar; 13(70): 193–9.

Ciacci C, Siniscalchi M, Bucci C, et al. Life events and the onset of celiac disease from a patient's perspective. *Nutrients*. 2013 Aug 28; 5(9): 3388–98.

Barouki R, Gluckman PD, Grandjean P, et al. Developmental origins of non-communicable disease: implications for research and public health. *Environ Health*. 2012 Jun 27; 11: 42.

Dietert RR. Developmental immunotoxicity, perinatal programming, and non-communicable diseases: focus on human studies. *Adv Med*. 2014 Jan; article ID 867805, 18 pages.

www.wheatbellyblog.com/2011/07/who-is-dr-william-davis.

Kasarda DD. Can an increase in celiac disease be attributed to an increase in the gluten content of wheat as a consequence of wheat breeding? *J Agric Food Chem*. 2013 Feb 13; 61(6): 1155–9.

Goddard CJ, Gillett HR. Complications of coeliac disease: are all patients at risk? *Postgrad Med J*. 2006 Nov; 82(973): 705–12.

Ludvigsson J, Bai J, Biagi F, et al. Guidelines: diagnosis and management of adult coeliac disease: guidelines from the British Society of Gastroenterology. *Gut*. 2014 Jun; doi: 10.1136/gutjnl-2013–306578.

Bürgin-Wolff A, Mauro B, Faruk H. Intestinal biopsy is not always required to diagnose celiac disease: a retrospective analysis of combined antibody tests. *BMC Gastroenterol*. 2013 Jan 23; 13: 19.

Thompson T. Gluten contamination of commercial oat products in the United States. *N Engl J Med*. 2004 Nov 4; 351(19): 2021–2.

Thompson T, Lee AR, Grace T. Gluten contamination of grains, seeds, and flours in the United States: a pilot study. *J Am Diet Assoc*. 2010 Jun; 110(6): 937–40.

Sbarbati A, Valletta E, Bertini M, et al. Gluten sensitivity and "normal" histology: is the intestinal mucosa really normal? *Dig Liver Dis*. 2003 Nov; 35(11): 768–73.

Cooper BT, Holmes GK, Ferguson R, et al. Gluten-sensitive diarrhea without evidence of celiac disease. *Gastroenterol*. 1980 Nov; 79(5 Pt 1): 801–6.

Catassi C, Bai JC, Bonaz B, et al. Non-celiac gluten sensitivity: the new frontier of gluten related disorders. *Nutrients*. Oct 2013; 5(10): 3839–53.

Sapone A, Bai JC, Ciacci C, et al. Spectrum of gluten-related disorders: consensus on new nomenclature and classification. *BMC Med*. 2012 Feb 7; 10: 13.

Nijeboer P, Bontkes HJ, Mulder CJ, et al. Non-celiac gluten sensitivity. Is it in the gluten or the grain? *J Gastrointestin Liver Dis*. 2013 Dec; 22(4): 435–40.

Corrao G, Corazza GR, Bagnardi V, et al. Mortality in patients with coeliac disease and their relatives: a cohort study. *Lancet*. 2001 Aug 4; 358(9279): 356–61.

Bartley J, McGlashan SR. Does milk increase mucus production? *Med Hypotheses*. 2010 Apr; 74(4): 732–4.

Azzouz A, Jurado-Sánchez B, Souhail B, et al. Simultaneous determination of 20 pharmacologically active substances in cow's milk, goat's milk, and human breast milk by gas chromatography-mass spectrometry. *J Agric Food Chem.* 2011 May 11; 59(9): 5125–32.

Schecter A, Haffner D, Colacino J, et al. Polybrominated diphenyl ethers (PBDEs) and hexabromocyclodecane (HBCD) in composite U.S. food samples. *Environ Health Perspect.* 2010 Mar; 118(3): 357–62.

Schecter A, Cramer P, Boggess K, et al. Intake of dioxins and related compounds from food in the U.S. population. *J Toxicol Environ Health A.* 2001 May 11; 63(1): 1–18.

Aris A, Leblanc S. Maternal and fetal exposure to pesticides associated to genetically modified foods in Eastern Townships of Quebec, Canada. *Reprod Toxicol.* 2011 May; 31(4): 528–33.

Choi YK, Kraft N, Zimmerman B, et al. Fructose intolerance in IBS and utility of fructose-restricted diet. *J Clin Gastroenterol.* 2008 Mar; 42(3): 233–8.

Thuy S, Ladurner R, Volynets V, et al. Nonalcoholic fatty liver disease in humans is associated with increased plasma endotoxin and plasminogen activator inhibitor 1 concentrations and with fructose intake. *J Nutr.* 2008 Aug; 138(8): 1452–5.

Frazier TH, DiBaise JK, McClain CJ. Gut microbiota, intestinal permeability, obesity-induced inflammation, and liver injury. *JPEN J Parenter Enteral Nutr.* 2011 Sep; 35(5 Suppl): 14S–20S.

Vos MB, Lavine JE. Dietary fructose in nonalcoholic fatty liver disease. *Hepatology.* 2013 Jun; 57(6): 2525–31.

Bøhn T, Cuhra M, Traavik T, et al. Compositional differences in soybeans on the market: glyphosate accumulates in Roundup Ready GM soybeans. *Food Chem.* 2014 Jun 15; 153: 207–15.

Padgette SR, Taylor NB, Nida DL, et al. The composition of glyphosate-tolerant soybean seeds is equivalent to that of conventional soybeans. *J Nutr.* 1996 Mar; 126(3): 702–16.

Darlington LG, Ramsey NW, Mansfield JR. Placebo-controlled, blind study of dietary manipulation therapy in rheumatoid arthritis. *Lancet.* 1986; 1: 236–8.

Hicklin JA, McEwen LM, Morgan JE. The effect of diet in rheumatoid arthritis. *Clin Allergy* 1980; 10: 463.

Zar S, Benson MJ, Kumar D. Food-specific serum IgG4 and IgE titers to common food antigens in irritable bowel syndrome. *Am J Gastroenterol.* 2005 Jul; 100(7): 1550–7.

Zar S, Mincher L, Benson MJ, et al. Food-specific IgG4 antibody-guided exclusion diet improves symptoms and rectal compliance in irritable bowel syndrome. *Scand J Gastroenterol.* 2005 Jul; 40(7): 800–7.

Granito A, Zauli D, Muratori P, et al. Anti-*Saccharomyces cerevisiae* and perinuclear anti-neutrophil cytoplasmic antibodies in coeliac disease before and after gluten-free diet. *Aliment Pharmacol Ther.* 2005 Apr 1; 21(7): 881–7.

Chapter 4

Policy statement—chemical-management policy: prioritizing children's health. Council on Environmental Health. *Pediatrics peds.* 2011–0523; published ahead of print April 25, 2011, doi: 10.1542/peds.2011–0523.

Casals-Casas C, Desvergne B. Endocrine disruptors: from endocrine to metabolic disruption. *Annu Rev Physiol.* 2011; 73: 135–62.

Genuis SJ, Sears M, Schwalfenberg G, et al. Incorporating environmental health in clinical medicine. *J Environ Public Health.* 2012; 2012: article ID 103041. Epub 2012 May 17.

Genuis SJ. What's out there making us sick? *J Environ Public Health.* 2012; 2012: article ID 605137. Epub 2011 Oct 24.

Grandjean P, Landrigan PJ. Neurobehavioural effects of developmental toxicity. *Lancet Neurol.* 2014 Mar; 13(3): 330–8.

Genuis SJ. Sensitivity-related illness: the escalating pandemic of allergy, food intolerance and chemical sensitivity. *Sci Total Environ.* 2010 Nov 15; 408(24): 6047–61.

Shehata AA, Schrödl W, Aldin AA, Hafez HM, Kruger M. The effect of glyphosate on potential pathogens and beneficial members of poultry microbiota in vitro. *Curr Microbiol.* 2013; 66 (4): 350–8.

Krüger M, Shehata AA, Schrödl W, Rodloff A. Glyphosate suppresses the antagonistic effect of *Enterococcus* spp. on *Clostridium botulinum. Anaerobe.* 2013; 20: 74–8.

Pascussi JM, Robert A, Nguyen M, et al. Possible involvement of pregnane X receptor-enhanced CYP24 expression in drug-induced osteomalacia. *J Clin Invest.* 2005 Jan; 115(1): 177–86.

Holick MF. Stay tuned to PXR: an orphan actor that may not be D-structive only to bone. *J Clin Invest.* 2005 Jan; 115(1): 32–4.

Kojima H, Sata F, Takeuchi S, et al. Comparative study of human and mouse pregnane X receptor agonistic activity in 200 pesticides using in vitro reporter gene assays. *Toxicol.* 2011 Feb 27; 280(3): 77–87.

Yang JH, Lee YM, Bae SG, et al. Associations between organochlorine pesticides and vitamin D deficiency in the U.S. population. *PLoS One.* 2012; 7(1): e30093.

Antico A, Tampoia M, Tozzoli R, et al. Can supplementation with vitamin D reduce the risk or modify the course of autoimmune diseases? A systematic review of the literature. *Autoimmun Rev.* 2012 Dec; 12(2): 127–36.

Hossein-nezhad A, Holick MF. Vitamin D for health: a global perspective. *Mayo Clin Proc.* 2013 Jul; 88(7): 720–55.

Kuo CH, Hsieh CC, Lee MS, et al. Epigenetic regulation in allergic diseases and related studies. *Asia Pac Allergy.* 2014 Jan; 4(1): 14–8.

Vogel SA. The politics of plastics: the making and unmaking of bisphenol A "safety." *Am J Public Health.* 2009 Nov; 99 Suppl 3: S559–66.

Vandenberg LN. Non-monotonic dose responses in studies of endocrine disrupting chemicals: bisphenol A as a case study. *Dose Response.* 2013 Oct 7; 12(2): 259–76.

Testa C, Nuti F, Hayek J, et al. Di-(2-ethylhexyl) phthalate and autism spectrum disorders. *ASN Neuro.* 2012 May 30; 4(4): 223–9.

Duty SM, Ackerman RM, Calafat AM, et al. Personal care product use predicts urinary concentrations of some phthalate monoesters. *Environ Health Perspect.* 2005 Nov; 113(11): 1530–5.

Genuis SJ, Beesoon S, Lobo RA, et al. Human elimination of phthalate compounds: blood, urine, and sweat (BUS) study. *Scientific World J.* 2012; 2012: article ID 615068.

Rudel RA, Gray JM, Engel CL, et al. Food packaging and bisphenol A and bis(2-ethyhexyl) phthalate exposure: findings from a dietary intervention. *Environ Health Perspect.* 2011 Jul; 119(7): 914–20.

Sexton K, Salinas JJ, McDonald TJ, et al. Biomarker measurements of prenatal exposure to polychlorinated biphenyls (PCB) in umbilical cord blood from postpartum Hispanic women in Brownsville, Texas. *J Toxicol Environ Health A.* 2013; 76(22): 1225–35.

Lee DH, Lee IK, Song K, et al. A strong dose-response relation between serum concentrations of persistent organic pollutants and diabetes: results from the National Health and Examination Survey 1999–2002. *Diabetes Care.* 2006 Jul; 29(7): 1638–44.

www.ewg.org/news/news-releases/2003/07/30/first-ever-us-tests-farmed-salmon-show-high-levels-cancer-causing-pcbs.

Choi YJ, Seelbach MJ, Pu H, et al. Polychlorinated biphenyls disrupt intestinal integrity via NADPH oxidase-induced alterations of tight junction protein expression. *Environ Health Perspect.* 2010 Jul; 118(7): 976–81.

www.akaction.org/Publications/Coal_Development/Toxic_Trade_Map_poster_mercury_final_8x10.pdf.

Qiu J. Tough talk over mercury treaty. *Nature.* 2013 Jan 10; 493(7431): 144–5.

http://www.briloon.org/uploads/BRI_Documents/Mercury_Center/BRI-IPEN-report-update-102214%20for%20web.pdf.

www.nbcnews.com/id/27704012/ns/world_news-world_environment/t/brown-clouds-dim-asia-threaten-worlds-food/#.U7D2RdxhfRo.

Savage JH, Matsui EC, Wood RA, et al. Urinary levels of triclosan and parabens are associated with aeroallergen and food sensitization. *J Allergy Clin Immunol.* 2012 Aug; 130(2): 453–60.e7.

Schab DW, Trinh NH. Do artificial food colors promote hyperactivity in children with hyperactive syndromes? A meta-analysis of double-blind placebo-controlled trials. *J Dev Behav Pediatr.* 2004 Dec; 25(6): 423–34.

Arnold LE, Lofthouse N, Hurt E. Artificial food colors and attention-deficit/hyperactivity symptoms: conclusions to dye for. *Neurotherapeutics.* 2012 Jul; 9(3): 599–609.

Jacobson MF. Carcinogenicity and regulation of caramel colorings. *Int J Occup Environ Health.* 2012 Jul-Sep; 18(3): 254–9.

Medeiros Vinci R, De Meulenaer B, Andjelkovic M, et al. Factors influencing benzene formation from the decarboxylation of benzoate in liquid model systems. *J Agric Food Chem*. 2011 Dec 28; 59(24): 12975–81.

Bendig P, Maier L, Lehnert K, et al. Mass spectra of methyl esters of brominated fatty acids and their presence in soft drinks and cocktail syrups. *Rapid Commun Mass Spectrom*. 2013 May 15; 27(9): 1083–9.

Bendig P, Maier L, Vetter W. Brominated vegetable oil in soft drinks—an underrated source of human organobromine intake. *Food Chem*. 2012; 133: 678.

Israel B, et al. Brominated battle: soda chemical has cloudy health history. *Scientific American*. Dec. 11, 2011. www.scientificamerican.com/article.cfm?id =soda-chemical-cloudy-health-history.

Horowitz BZ. Bromism from excessive cola consumption. *J Toxicol Clin Toxicol*. 1997; 35(3): 315–20.

Jih DM, Khanna V, Somach SC. Bromoderma after excessive ingestion of Ruby Red Squirt. *N Engl J Med*. 2003 May 8; 348(19): 1932–4.

ntp.niehs.nih.gov/ntp/roc/twelfth/profiles/butylatedhydroxyanisole.pdf.

Vandenberg LN, Colborn T, Hayes TB, et al. Regulatory decisions on endocrine disrupting chemicals should be based on the principles of endocrinology. *Reprod Toxicol*. 2013 Jul; 38: 1–15.

Vandenberg LN. Non-monotonic dose responses in studies of endocrine disrupting chemicals: bisphenol A as a case study. *Dose Response*. 2013 Oct 7; 12(2): 259–76.

Vandenberg LN, Colborn T, Hayes TB, et al. Hormones and endocrine-disrupting chemicals: low-dose effects and nonmonotonic dose responses. *Endocr Rev*. 2012 Jun; 33(3): 378–455.

big.assets.huffingtonpost.com/fraud.pdf.

Cattani D, de Liz Oliveira Cavalli VL, Heinz Rieg CE, et al. Mechanisms underlying the neurotoxicity induced by glyphosate-based herbicide in immature rat hippocampus: involvement of glutamate excitotoxicity. *Toxicol*. 2014 Jun 5; 320: 34–45.

Jayasumana C, Gunatilake S, Senanayake P, et al. Glyphosate, hard water and nephrotoxic metals: are they the culprits behind the epidemic of chronic kidney disease of unknown etiology in Sri Lanka? *Int J Environ Res Public Health*. 2014; 11(2): 2125–47.

Lushchak OV, Kubrak OI, Storey JM, et al. Low toxic herbicide Roundup induces mild oxidative stress in goldfish tissues. *Chemosphere*. 2009 Aug; 76(7): 932–7.

De Liz Oliveira Cavalli VL, Cattani D, Heinz Rieg CE, et al. Roundup disrupts male reproductive functions by triggering calcium-mediated cell death in rat testis and Sertoli cells. *Free Radic Biol Med*. 2013 Dec; 65: 335–46.

Shehata AA, Schrödl W, Aldin AA, et al. The effect of glyphosate on potential pathogens and beneficial members of poultry microbiota in vitro. *Curr Microbiol*. 2013 Apr; 66(4): 350–8.

Séralini GE, Mesnage R, Clair E, et al. Genetically modified crops safety assessments: present limits and possible improvements. *Environ Sci Europe*. 2011 Mar 1; 23: 10.

Paganelli A, Gnazzo V, Acosta H, et al. Glyphosate-based herbicides produce teratogenic effects on vertebrates by impairing retinoic acid signaling. *Chem Res Toxicol*. 2010 Aug 9; 23(10): 1586–95.

El-Shenawy NS. Oxidative stress responses of rats exposed to Roundup and its active ingredient glyphosate. *Environ Toxicol Pharmacol*. 2009 Nov; 28(3): 379–85.

Gui YX, Fan XN, Wang HM, et al. Glyphosate induced cell death through apoptotic and autophagic mechanisms. *Neurotoxicol Teratol*. 2012; 34: 344–9.

patft.uspto.gov/netacgi/nph-Parser?Sect1=PTO2&Sect2=HITOFF&p=1&u=/netahtml/PTO/search-bool.html&r=1&f=G&l=50&co1=AND&d=PTXT&s1=7771736.PN.&OS=PN/7771736&RS=PN/7771736.

Krüger M, Schledorn P, Schrödl W, et al. Detection of glyphosate residues in animals and humans. *J Environ Anal Toxicol*. 2014 Jan; 4: 2.

Krüger M, Shehata AA, Schrödl W, et al. Glyphosate suppresses the antagonistic effect of *Enterococcus* spp. on *Clostridium botulinum*. *Anaerobe*. 2013 Apr; 20: 74–8.

www.biointegrity.org/

sustainablepulse.com/wp-content/uploads/GMO-health.pdf.

www.examiner.com/article/connect-the-dots-2.

Zobiole LH, Kremer RJ, Oliveira RS Jr, et al. Glyphosate affects micro-organisms in rhizospheres of glyphosate-resistant soybeans. *J Appl Microbiol*. 2011 Jan; 110(1): 118–27.

Mesnage R, Bernay B, Séralini GE. Ethoxylated adjuvants of glyphosate-based herbicides are active principles of human cell toxicity. *Toxicol*. 2013 Nov 16; 313(2–3): 122–8.

Mesnage R, Defarge N, Spiroux de Vendômois J, et al. Major pesticides are more toxic to human cells than their declared active principles. *Biomed Res Int*. 2014; 2014: article ID 179691.

Brandt K, Leifert C, Sanderson R, et al. Agroecosystem management and nutritional quality of plant foods: the case of organic fruits and vegetables. *Crit Rev Plant Sci*. 2011; 30: 177–97.

Smith-Spangler C, Brandeau ML, Hunter GE, et al. Are organic foods safer or healthier than conventional alternatives? A systematic review. *Ann Intern Med*. 2012 Sep 4; 157(5): 348–66.

Benbrook C. Are organic foods safer or healthier? *Ann Intern Med*. 2013 Feb 19; 158(4): 296–97.

Lu C, Toepel K, Irish R, et al. Organic diets significantly lower children's dietary exposure to organophosphorus pesticides. *Environ Health Perspect*. 2006 Feb; 114(2): 260–3.

Roberts EM, English PB, Grether JK, et al. Maternal residence near agricultural pesticide applications and autism spectrum disorders among children in the California Central Valley. *Environ Health Perspect.* 2007 Oct; 115(10): 1482–9.

Shelton JF, Geraghty EM, Tancredi DJ, et al. Neurodevelopmental disorders and prenatal residential proximity to agricultural pesticides: the CHARGE study. *Environ Health Perspect.* 2014 Jun 23. [Epub ahead of print].

healthland.time.com/2011/04/21/exposure-to-pesticides-in-pregnancy-can-lower-childrens-iq.

Chapter 5

Hossein-nezhad A, Holick MF. Vitamin D for health: a global perspective. *Mayo Clin Proc.* 2013 Jul; 88(7): 720–55.

Rosanoff A, Weaver CM, Rude RK. Suboptimal magnesium status in the United States: are the health consequences underestimated? *Nutr Rev.* 2012 Mar; 70(3): 153–64.

Chacko SA, Sul J, Song Y, et al. Magnesium supplementation, metabolic and inflammatory markers, and global genomic and proteomic profiling: a randomized, double-blind, controlled, crossover trial in overweight individuals. *Am J Clin Nutr.* 2011 Feb; 93(2): 463–73.

Zhang Y, Talalay P, Cho CG, et al. A major inducer of anticarcinogenic protective enzymes from broccoli: isolation and elucidation of structure. *Proc Natl Acad Sci USA.* 1992 Mar 15; 89(6): 2399–403.

Yamamoto M, Singh A, Sava F, et al. MicroRNA expression in response to controlled exposure to diesel exhaust: attenuation by the antioxidant N-acetylcysteine in a randomized crossover study. *Environ Health Perspect.* 2013 Jun; 121(6): 670–5.

Gomes AC, Bueno AA, de Souza RG, et al. Gut microbiota, probiotics and diabetes. *Nutr J.* 2014 Jun 17; 13(1): 60.

Han J, Lin H, Huang W. Modulating gut microbiota as an anti-diabetic mechanism of berberine. *Med Sci Monit.* 2011 Jul; 17(7): RA164–7.

Di Pierro F, Rapacioli G, Di Maio EA, et al. Comparative evaluation of the pain-relieving properties of a lecithinized formulation of curcumin (Meriva(®)), nimesulide, and acetaminophen. *J Pain Res.* 2013; 6: 201–5.

Belcaro G, Cesarone MR, Dugall M, et al. Efficacy and safety of Meriva®, a curcumin-phosphatidylcholine complex, during extended administration in osteoarthritis patients. *Altern Med Rev.* 2010 Dec; 15(4): 337–44.

Chapter 6

Rustagi N, Pradhan SK, Singh R. Public health impact of plastics: an overview. *Indian J Occup Environ Med.* 2011 Sep; 15(3): 100–3.

Chapter 7

Demmig-Adams B, Adams WW III. Antioxidants in photosynthesis and human nutrition. *Science.* 2002 Dec 13; 298(5601): 2149–53. PMID: 12481128.

Subbiah MT. Understanding the nutrigenomic definitions and concepts at the food-genome junction. *OMICS.* 2008 Dec; 12(4): 229–35. PMID: 18687041.

Hanhineva K, Törrönen R, Bondia-Pons I, et al. Impact of dietary polyphenols on carbohydrate metabolism. *Int J Mol Sci.* 2010 Mar 31; 11(4): 1365–402. PMID: 20480025.

Park WT, Kim JK, Park S, et al. Metabolic profiling of glucosinolates, anthocyanins, carotenoids, and other secondary metabolites in kohlrabi (*Brassica oleracea* var. *gongylodes*). *J Agric Food Chem.* 2012 Jun 28. [Epub ahead of print].

Mikaili P, Maadirad S, Moloudizargari M, et al. Therapeutic uses and pharmacological properties of garlic, shallot, and their biologically active compounds. *Iran J Basic Med Sci.* 2013 Oct; 16(10): 1031–48.

Sehitoglu MH, Farooqi AA, Qureshi MZ, et al. Anthocyanins: targeting of signaling networks in cancer cells. *Asian Pac J Cancer Prev.* 2014; 15(5): 2379–81.

Xie M, Nghiem LD, Price WE, et al. Comparison of the removal of hydrophobic trace organic contaminants by forward osmosis and reverse osmosis. *Water Res.* 2012 May 15; 46(8): 2683–92.

www.sciencedaily.com/releases/2012/08/120820143902.htm (accessed July 3, 2014).

Chapter 8

Lasky T, Sun W, Kadry A, et al. Mean total arsenic concentrations in chicken 1989–2000 and estimated exposures for consumers of chicken. *Environ Health Perspect.* 2004 Jan; 112(1): 18–21. PMID: 14698925.

Silbergeld EK, Nachman K. The environmental and public health risks associated with arsenical use in animal feeds. *Ann N Y Acad Sci.* 2008 Oct; 1140: 346–57. PMID: 18991934.

Harris, G, Grady, D. Pfizer suspends sales of chicken drug with arsenic. June 8, 2011. NewYorkTimes.com. Retrieved on March 16, 2012, from www.nytimes.com/2011/06/09/business/09arsenic.html?_r=3.

Han JR, Deng B, Sun J, et al. Effects of dietary medium-chain triglyceride on weight loss and insulin sensitivity in a group of moderately overweight free-living type 2 diabetic Chinese subjects. *Metabolism.* 2007 Jul; 56(7): 985–91. PMID: 17570262.

Kasai M, Nosaka N, Maki H, et al. Effect of dietary medium- and long-chain triacylglycerols (MLCT) on accumulation of body fat in healthy humans. *Asia Pac J Clin Nutr.* 2003; 12(2): 151–60. PMID: 12810404.

St-Onge MP, Bosarge A. Weight-loss diet that includes consumption of medium-chain triacylglycerol oil leads to a greater rate of weight and fat mass loss than does olive oil. *Am J Clin Nutr.* 2008 Mar; 87(3): 621–6. PMID: 18326600.

Chapter 9

Corrao G, Corazza GR, Bagnardi V, et al. Mortality in patients with coeliac disease and their relatives: a cohort study. *Lancet*. 2001 Aug 4; 358(9279): 356–61.

Ludvigsson JF, Montgomery SM, Ekbom A, et al. Small-intestinal histopathology and mortality risk in celiac disease. *JAMA*. 2009 Sep 16; 302(11): 1171–8.

Chapter 10

Williams BL, Hornig M, Buie T, et al. Impaired carbohydrate digestion and transport and mucosal dysbiosis in the intestines of children with autism and gastrointestinal disturbances. *PLOS One*. 2011; 6(9):e24585. doi: 10.1371/journal.pone .0024585. Epub 2011 Sep 16.

INDEX

bacteria, beneficial, 39, 41–42, 52, 73, 74, 106, 297. *See also* probiotics
banana muffins, 225
barley, 18, 20, 21, 49, 153, 172, 181
basil-radish quinoa salad, 249
bath. *See* Epsom salt bath
beans, 167, 180, 181. *See also specific types*
beef, 64
    elimination, 27, 1887
    reintroduction, 170, 173, 200, 220
beef stew, nightshade-free, 220–21
beer, 49, 63, 153
beets
    fennel juice, 191–92
    rosemary detox soup, 299
beet sugar, 85, 156
belching, prevention, 32
berberine, 112, 167, 183
berries, 22, 104, 181
    smoothies, 192–96
    vanilla milkshake, 195
    with whipped vanilla coconut cream, 280
betaine HCL, 33, 34, 143, 167, 183
beverages, 127, 129–32, 153–54, 184
    recipes, 289–94
biocide, 73, 82
bisphenol-A (BPA), 75, 115
black bean:
    quinoa dosas, 222–23
    yam, and avocado tacos, 255–56
black tea, 153, 170, 184
blender, high-powered, 104
bloating, 10, 22, 27, 29, 33, 36, 48, 54, 56, 58, 61, 65, 106, 112, 113, 128, 165, 182, 186
    causes, 31
    prevention, 32, 47
    reintroduced foods, 167, 169, 180
blood test markers, 54–55, 56
blueberries, 104
    vinaigrette, 231, 272
bowel movement, 4, 10, 11, 13, 22, 36, 37, 49, 50, 106, 112, 113, 139, 165, 186
    digestive enzymes test, 39
    fructose malabsorption, 61, 62
    leaky gut syndrome symptom, 44
    magnesium supplement, 108–9
    reintroduced foods, 169, 180
    See also constipation; diarrhea
Brazil nuts, 195, 197

bread:
    alternatives, 222–23, 227–28, 267, 270
    craving, 179
    gluten content, 49
breakfast recipes, 198–205
breast milk. *See* lactation
breathing problems, 4, 13–14, 19, 169
broccoli, 105, 110, 129, 146, 188
    creamy mushroom soup, 208–9
broccoli sprouts, 76, 78, 105–6, 129, 179, 184
    detoxification qualities, 110
    growing from seed, 106, 301–2
brominated vegetable oil (BVO), 80
broth recipes, 216, 218
Brown Cloud, 77
brown rice, 144, 181, 182
    adzuki bean salad, 248–49
    basic recipe, 246
    creamy cereal, 198
    flour, 225, 228
    mung bean kitcheree, 252–53
    tortillas, 223–24
    vegetable nori rolls, 250–51
Brussels sprouts, 105, 110, 129, 188
    roasted with cauliflower, 242
buckwheat, 145
burgers:
    chicken-spinach, 263
    mustard-herb lamb, 270
butcher shop, 118
butternut squash, sage stuffing, 239–40
butters, 157, 241, 281, 283, 284–85
butylated hydroxyanisole (BHA), 80
butylated hydroxytoluent (BHT), 80

cabbage, 105, 129
    berry smoothie, 193
    chicken soup, 214
    rainbow kraut, 299–300
    salad with ginger cilantro dressing, 232–34
    See also sauerkraut
caffeine:
    breast milk effect, 188
    craving, 179, 184
    elimination, 131, 142, 153, 156, 184
calcium, 83, 108, 149
    deficiency, 33
calories, 27
cancer, 74, 75, 80, 104, 105, 112, 129

immunoglobulins. *See* IgA antibodies;
    IgE antibodies
indigestion, 32–35
inflammation, 6–7, 19, 20, 24–26, 29, 37, 48,
    73, 129, 177–78, 293
    chemicals, 50–51, 66
    chronic, 24, 25, 41, 45, 53
    reduction, 112, 165
    symptoms, 141
    system-wide, 17
    triggers, 25
    uncontrolled, 125
inflammatory bowel disease, 112, 182
insomnia. *See* sleep problems
intestinal lining, *40*
    celiac attack on, 53
    cell layer, 35–36, 42–43
    damaging substances, 43, 51, 182–83
    permeability. *See* leaky gut syndrome
iodine, 211
irritable bowel syndrome, 4, 39, 62, 74, 84,
    112, 141, 182

jasmine rice, 181
joint pain, 6, 17, 22, 23, 24, 44, 48, 54, 57, 109,
    141, 142, 145, 165
    easing of, 99, 104
    reintroduced foods, 166, 169
journal keeping, 27, 95–98, 125, 139, 168–69
    sample page, 97–98
juices, 190–92, 220, 260. *See also* vegetable
    juice

kabocha squash, 107, 146, 219, 220, 241
kale, 105, 129, 145, 179, 188, 205
    chickpea curry with potatoes, 254–55
    chips, salt and pepper, 244–45
    cleansing juice, 190
    salad with lemon and garlic, 235–36
    sautéed with shiitake mushrooms, 239
    smoothie, 194
    sweet potato hash, 200–201
    turkey and carrot hash, 199–200
    white bean, wild rice soup, 212–13
    zucchini and egg scramble, 203
kefir, 106
kitchen, 114–21
    Elimination Diet essentials, 295–302
    equipment upgrade, 114–16

kitchen garden, 104–5
    broccoli sprouts, 106, 301–2
    herbs, 117, 151
kombucha, 185, 297

lactase enzyme, 21, 58
lactation, 59, 187–88
lactose, 181
lactose intolerance, 21, 22
    symptoms, 58
lamb
    mustard-herb burgers, 270
    quinoa breakfast hash, 201–2
large intestine, 30, 39–40
leaky gut syndrome (LGS), 25, 30, 35, 44–51,
    52, 53, 57, 61, 62, 64, 67, 76
    cause, 43, 48–51, 59, 293
    symptoms, 44
lectins, 35–36, 44, 57
leeks
    cauliflower and lemon salad, 338
    chopping tip, 206
leftovers, 116
legumes, 156, 187
    elimination, 181, 182
lemon
    cauliflower and leek salad, 238
    garnish, 258
    juice, 276
    raw kale salad with garlic, 235–36
    salad dressing, 271–72, 273
lettuce, 145
    romaine salad, 234–35
    wraps, 267, 270
lime, 170, 172, 175, 187, 194, 195, 219, 220,
    229, 250
liver, 36, 61, 110

magnesium, 108–9, 146
    deficiency signs, 33, 109
main meal recipes, 252–70
manganese, 83, 149
mangoes, 62, 181
maple syrup, 148, 149, 157, 182
meal plans, 137, 158–62, 172–76
meatballs, turkey-herb-quinoa, 268–69
meats
    elimination, 154
    fermented, 106

peach-coconut milk creamsicles, 187–88
peanuts, 27, 66–67, 188
    allergy, 20
    reintroduction, 171, 174–75
pears, 62, 180, 181
pecans, 171, 174, 240
peppers, 170, 188, 201, 202, 235
peptides, 43, 50, 183
persistent organic pollutants (POPs), 59
personal care items, 75, 166
pesticides and herbicides, 25, 41, 45, 47, 60,
    62, 63, 68, 71, 73–74, 81–88, 146
phenols, 21, 22, 75, 147
Phillips' Colon Health, 111
pH level, 31–32, 33
phthalates, 75–76, 116
phytates, 67
phytochemicals, 128–29, 146, 154
pickles, 106, 297–99
pineapple, 104
    green smoothie, 194–95
pistachios, 171, 181
plastic, 75, 76
plastic-free utensils, 115, 116
pollen, 25
pollutants. See environmental chemicals
polychlorinated biphenyls. See PCBs
pomegranate chicken tacos, 259–60
pomegranate juice, 220, 260
pork, 27, 64, 171, 173
postnasal drip, 13, 22
potassium, 149
potatoes, 187
    chickpea curry with kale, 254–55
prebiotics, 42, 149
pregnancy, 72, 75, 76, 187
preservatives, 21, 73, 79, 80, 153
prick test reliability, 20
probiotics, 42, 106, 111, 187, 277, 297
processed foods, 17, 41, 145, 186–87
    "gluten-free" products, 55
    gluten in, 49, 52
    soy additive, 62
prolamins, 60
protease inhibitors, 59
protein, 19, 31, 49, 58, 66–67, 142–44
    allergic reaction, 20
    carbohydrate-binding, 44
    lectins, 35–36

undigested, 59
    zonulin, 44, 51
psoriasis, 14, 53, 169
pumpkin pie chia pudding, 286–87
pumpkin seeds
    delicata squash salad with apples, 231–32
    energy bars, 282–83
    spiced granola, 204–5
    toasting tip, 233
purified water, 127, 129, 130, 153, 289

quinoa, 144, 181, 182
    basic recipe, 247–48
    basil salad, 249
    black bean dosas, 222–23
    coconut breakfast porridge, 198–99
    cucumber-dill salad, 250
    lamb breakfast hash, 201
    turkey-herb meatballs, 268–69

radishes, 105, 110, 179
    spring salad with snap peas and salmon,
        230
rash. See skin problems
RAST test reliability, 20
raw honey, 148, 149, 157, 182, 184, 197, 225,
    227
Raynaud's disease, 54
reactive foods, 48–69
recipes, 189–302
    Phase 1, 138
    Phase 2, 162–64
    Phase 3, 170, 176–77
red bell pepper, 201, 202, 235
red cabbage, 129
    berry smoothie, 193
reintroduction (Phase 3), 27, 125, 165–78
    challenges, 166–69, 180–85, 258–59
    meal plan, 172–76
    recipes, 170, 176–77
    schedule, 169–72, 220–21, 267
rheumatoid arthritis, 24, 44, 46, 54, 64
rice, 144, 182
    cereal, 198
    flour, 181
    pulsed cauliflower replacing, 260–61
    vinegar, 152
    See also brown rice; wild rice
romaine salad, Italian herb dressing, 234–35

ABOUT THE AUTHORS

ALISSA SEGERSTEN received her bachelor of science in nutrition from Bastyr University in Kenmore, Washington. She is the previous owner of a personal chef business in Seattle, Washington, through which she successfully addressed the health and lifestyle needs of many families with her delicious, healthy cooking. She is a full-time mother to her five children and enjoys organic gardening, food preservation, wild-harvesting food, and hiking in the mountains with her family. She is currently a cooking instructor through her live classes and online programs, empowering people with cooking skills and knowledge of whole foods so that they may reconnect with the pleasure in eating delicious, nourishing food. Her popular recipe blog, NourishingMeals.com, is filled with healthy, wholesome, gluten-free recipes.

TOM MALTERRE MS, CN, holds both a bachelor's and master's degree in nutrition from Bastyr University, has advanced training from the Institute for Functional Medicine, and has over a decade of clinical experience. Tom is a current faculty member of the Autism Research Institute and was a medical affairs member of Thorne Research. He has lectured on nutrition and supplementation across the United States and Canada. He currently coaches doctors and other health-care practitioners on Functional Medicine protocols in his Progressive Practitioner Coaching Programs, while doing interviews and blogging on a vast array of health topics. When he is not seeing clients or contemplating nutritional sciences, he can be found out in nature with his five children, wild-harvesting native plants, practicing archery, hiking, camping, and rock climbing.